MOTHERS AND DAUGHTERS:
The Real Physician to Daughters

PRACTICAL STUDIES

FOR THE CONSERVATION OF THE HEALTH OF GIRLS.

BY

TULLIO SUZZARA VERDI, A.M., M.D.

AUTHOR OF "MATERNITY
A TREATISE FOR YOUNG WIVES AND MOTHERS:"
PRESIDENT OF THE BOARD OF HEALTH,
WASHINGTON, D.C.; ETC.

"This hour's the very crisis of your fate."
—*Dryden.*

HEALTH 🌳 HARMONY

NOTE FROM THE PUBLISHERS

Any information given in this book is not intended to be taken as a replacement for medical advice. Any person with a condition requiring medical attention should consult a qualified practitioner or therapist.

© All rights are reserved. No part of this publication may be reproduced, stored in a retrieval system or transmitted, in any form or by any means, mechanical, photocopying, recording or otherwise, without prior written permission of the publishers.

Price: Rs. 80.00

First Edition, 1986

Reprint edition 2002

Published by

KULDEEP JAIN

for

HEALTH  **HARMONY**

1921, Chuna Mandi, St. 10th, Paharganj,
New Delhi-110 055
Ph: 3670430, 3670572, 3683200, 3683300
Fax: 011-3610471 & 3683400
Website: www.bjainbooks.com, Email: bjain@vsnl.com

Printed in India by
Unisons Techno Financial Consultants (P) Ltd.
522, FIE, Patpar Ganj, Delhi-110 092

ISBN : 81-7021-1107-0

BOOK CODE : BV-2796

CONTENTS.

PAGE

PREFACE.

PART I.

PHYSIOLOGY OF WOMEN.

CHAPTER I.
THE MOTHER'S DUTY.

The Mother's duty to her Daughter.—Responsibility of Parents and Teachers for the Girl's Ignorance of the Modes to Preserve her Health.—Relative Position of Man and Woman in their Struggle for Existence.—Disability of Girls for Work.—Triumph of Health and Strength. 7–15

CHAPTER II.
A VEXED QUESTION.

Importance of Studying the Body.—Distinctive Characteristics of the Sexes.—Physical Vigor the Foundation of Man's General Advantage. —Comparison of Man and Woman as Workers.—Soundness of Body Woman's Greatest Present Need 16–26

CHAPTER III.
PHYSIOLOGY AS A MORAL TEACHER.

What are Anatomy and Physiology.—Force.—Health.—Laws of Nature and their Infringement.—Responsibility of Man for the Infraction of Natural Laws.—Accident.—Sanitary Science and Disease.—Helplessness of Ignorance. 27–30

CHAPTER IV.
MORAL AND PHYSICAL CHARACTERISTICS OF THE TWO SEXES IN RELATION TO THEIR GROWTH AFTER PUBERTY.

Man's Strength, Woman's Heroism.—Illustrations.—Specific Differences of Physical Structure.—Adaptation of their Physical Nature to the Requirements of the Two Sexes 31–39

CHAPTER V.

THE PELVIS.

Anatomy of Woman's Pelvis, and its Mode of Growth.—Important Reflections.—Necessary Protection to the Pelvis of Little Girls.—Dangers of Deformed Pelvis from the Dressing of Infants and very Young Girls. 40–45

CHAPTER VI.

THE WOMB.

Anatomy of the Womb.—Manner of Growth. 46–48

CHAPTER VII.

FALLOPIAN TUBES AND OVARIES.

Anatomy of the Fallopian Tubes and Ovaries.—Their Functions and Relative Positions. 49–51

CHAPTER VIII.

THE MAMMÆ OR BREASTS.

Relations of these Organs to the Development of Beauty and Utility of Woman.—Anatomy of the Same.—How Dress Affects the Development of the Breasts.—Sympathy of the Breasts with the Generative Organs.—Necessity to Protect their Growth. 52–58

CHAPTER IX.

TEMPERAMENTS.

Temperaments as the Guide for Moral and Physical Education.—Description and Hygienic Requirements of the Sanguine, Lymphatic Bilious, Nervous, Mixed Temperaments.—Modification of the Temperaments by Climate, Education, Habits and Social Condition. . . 59–69

CHAPTER X.

PUBERTY.

The Four Periods of Life, Infancy, Adolescence, Virility, Dementia.—Development of Puberty in Woman.—Vital Importance of this Period.—Menstruation.—Warning Symptoms of the Approach of Puberty in Girls. 70–78

CHAPTER XI.

PHILOSOPHY AND PHYSIOLOGY OF MENSTRUATION.

Physiology of Menstruation and Mode of Appearance.—History of Menstruation.—Menstruation in Relation to Ovulation.—Ovulation.—Menstrual Crisis.—Epoch of its Commencement and Mode of its Course.—Northern and Southern Girls.—City and Country Girls.—Effect of Temperaments.—Periodical Calculations.—Specific Course of Menstruation 79–92

CONTENTS.

v

PART II

HYGIENE FOR WOMEN.

CHAPTER I.
HYGIENIC GENERALITIES.

Hygienic Generalities.—Light.—Heat.—Exercise.—A Warning to Mothers 95-99

CHAPTER II.
SOCIETY, IN ITS RELATION TO THE HEALTH OF GIRLS.

Communities.—Social Laws.—Fashion.—Dress.—Diet.—Amusements.—Exaggerations of Life.—Mme. George Sand's Lament.—How to Preserve the Health and Life of Woman 100-113

CHAPTER III.
EXERCISE AND ITS RELATION TO BODILY FUNCTIONS.

Physiological Effects of Exercise.—Excessive Exercise.—Adequate Rest.—Sedentary Life.—Modes of Exercise.—Walking.—Riding.—Dancing.—Rowing.—Games.—Passive Exercise.—Driving.—Sea-Going.—Singing.—Gymnastics 114-124

CHAPTER IV.
FOOD.

Its Relations to the Preservation of Life.—Digestion.—Assimilation.—Absorption.—Experiments of Dr. Beaumont.—Liebig's Division of Food in Classes.—History of Food.—Food and the Human Family.—Food and Civilization.—Physiology of Food.—Bad Digestion and Human Happiness.—Food and its Elements.—Direction for Kinds and Qualities of Food.—Classification of Food.—Time Required for Digesting Articles of Food.—Food Affecting Individual Character.—Rules for Diet. 125-149

CHAPTER V.
CLOTHING.

Its Lessons in the Preservation of Life.—Clothing and Climates.—Reasons for Clothing.—History of the Corset, and its Baneful Effects.—Materials for Clothing.—Articles of Clothing and their Heat Conducting Power.—Color in Relation to Dress.—Heat Conducting Power of Colors.—Clothing of Special Parts; Head, Neck, Trunk, Extremities.—Moisture, Malaria Prevented by Modes of Dressing.—Partial and General Dressing.—Partial Dressing a Cause of Disease.—How Dress May Affect Girls.—Constipation of Women Induced by Unphysiological Dressing of Young Girls.—"The Cowl Does not Make the Friar." 150-172

CHAPTER VI.

AIR.

Atmospheric Conditions in Relation to Human Health.—Hot and Dry, Cold and Dry, Damp and Hot, Cold and Humid.—Movement of the Air.—Mountain Air.—Sea Air.—Rapid Changes of Temperature.—Impure Air of Dwellings.—Cubic Feet of Pure Air for each Person.—Carbonic Acid in the Atmosphere of Dwelling and Schools.—Ventilation.—Air of Sleeping Rooms.—Combustion of Coal, Wood, Gas, Oil, Candles and the Carbonic Acid they Emit.—Atmosphere of Water-Closets, Bath-Rooms.—Sewage Gases Coming into Inhabited Rooms, How to Prevent it. 173–188

PART III.

FUNCTIONAL IRREGULARITIES, AND THEIR PREVENTIVE TREATMENT.

CHAPTER I.

SYMPTOMS OF DISTURBANCE.

Signs of Puberty.—Menstruation.—Colic.—Coldness of Feet.—Rest.—Dress.—Food and Drink.—Demeanor.—Different Temperaments.—Symptoms that may Occur 191–196

CHAPTER II.

CAUSES OF FUNCTIONAL DERANGEMENTS.

Indispositions of Girls During Menstruation.—Causes of Derangement of Uterine Functions.—Remote Causes.—Temperaments.—Diet.—Bad Air.—Want of Exercise.—Mind and Imagination.—Opinions of High Authorities Regarding School Exercises and Girls' Debility.—A Mother's Story of her Daughter's Death from too Close Application to Study.—Effects of Wet, Heat and Cold on Menstrual Functions.—Uncleanliness.—Dress.—Occupation.—Immediate Causes.—Exposures.—Emotions.—Accident and other Causes 197–217

CHAPTER III.

AMENORRHŒA.

Delayed Menstruation.—Suppression and Retention of the Menses.—Chlorosis.—Their Symptoms, Causes, Difference, and the Preventive Treatment. 218–233

CHAPTER IV.

MENORRHAGIA.

Excessive Menstruation.—Active, Passive, Nervous or Spasmodic.—Causes, Symptoms and Preventive Treatment. . . . 234–204

CONTENTS.

CHAPTER V.

DYSMENORRHŒA.

PAGE

Painful Menstruation.—Simple, Accidental, Congestive, Inflammatory, Mechanical Dysmenorrhœa.—Causes, Symptoms and Hygienic Treatment. 241-250

CHAPTER VI.

LEUCORRHŒA.

Whites.—Acute and Chronic.—Causes, Symptoms and Hygienic Treatment. 251-257

CHAPTER VII.

HYSTERIA.

Characteristics of Women Predisposed to it.—Predisposing Causes.—Immediate Causes ; Hysteria Simulating Other Diseases.—Illustrations.—Symptoms of Simple Hysteria.—Hygienic Treatment.—Education and Hysteria. 258-273

CHAPTER VIII.

INFLAMMATION AND DISPLACEMENTS OF THE WOMB.

Acute, and Chronic, Causes and Hygienic Treatment.—Displacements of the Uterus ; Prolapsus, Anteversion, Retroversion, Inversion, Procidentia.—Simple Displacements.—Causes, Symptoms and Hygienic Treatment. 274-281

PREFACE.

THERE was a time when medicine, or what was supposed to be the medical art, was the property of necromancers, or of high-priests who consulted the oracles. A tithe was paid for the oracle; the larger the tithe the more favorable the answer: and the wise men of those days anathematized all philosophers daring to get a peep at the works of nature.

We have the same wise men now, only not so bold, as human intelligence has risen above ignorance and superstition. Yet we have them; and they hold that medicine is their province, and that attempts made to induce the people to seek information in its realms are flagrant violations of their inherited and sacred rights.

But with the development of human intellect came a desire of independence which even these high-priests could not restrain. Thousands of learned physicians severed the chains of professional slavery to teach the people that the mystical philosophy of the physician is but the study of nature, which even the humblest citizen should have the privilege of enquiring into. These teachers are not condemned to the stake now

—civilization forbids it; but in the scarlet chambers where they hold council the high-priests condemn these humanitarians to the pillory of their scorn and to the denunciation of the faculty. The times are more auspicious, however; bigotry is daily loosening its grasp, and more physicians are now converted to faith in freedom than ever before.

Exclusiveness having heretofore been the practice of medical men, it is not surprising that the people remained ignorant of even the simplest rules for the preservation of their health. Under that system the functions of the human economy were, in polite society, a sort of forbidden ground, a discussion or a mention of which could not be tolerated. This unreasonable custom finally degenerated into prudery and false modesty. Woman, naturally more delicate-minded than man, under this social restraint became very reticent, and it was with difficulty that she would mention any organ of her body, even though she suffered general discomfort, and even great pain. The mother watched the roses fading on the cheeks of her daughter, and yet did not dare to ask for the causes that induced the apparent disturbance. It was only when disease became fully developed, or the girl had fallen into an extremity of debility, that the physician was called in, who would often find that neglect or diffidence had allowed a simple disorder to grow into a permanent disease.

These erroneous notions of propriety have largely contributed to the degeneracy of the health of girls, particularly in the higher spheres of social life.

In every household will be found young women who, from the day of their entrance upon womanhood, have become victims of periodical sufferings; mothers, who, after giving birth to a child or two, are exhausted for the remainder of their lives; women who drag a suffering body in the exercise of family duties.

The learned physician now looks upon these social customs and practices as the cause of the deterioration of women, drops the purely medical art—the drug, that cannot bring blood to their arteries, tissue to their muscles, or bone to their frames—and studies the organization of their nature and the requirements for its preservation. The Hygeia of antiquity was a mythological idea; Hygiene of to-day is a science. It is the science that teaches how to conduct, how to preserve life; it is not the art of curing disease, it is the science of preventing it. Shall we keep it from the young, who have a life to preserve, to offer it to the old, whose life's thread has passed from Clotho to Lachesis, and is already held by Atropos the inexorable?

Invalidism prevails amongst the women of our generation. This fact should concern not only the physician, but the statesman, the political economist and the lover of mankind. Has the civilization of the last century done no more for woman than to reduce her strength and her capacity? If so, it is high time that it direct its best efforts to her moral and physical improvement. Is not the present system of female education founded upon a radical error, when it is proven by statistical observations that the physical condition of the educated woman is far inferior to that of her illiterate laboring sister? Parents should reflect upon this fact so often stated and reasserted by every medical authority.

Education cannot imperil the life of a student if in the curriculum of her studies the science to preserve her life is included. In every school there should be taught anatomy, physiology and hygiene—and the latter *practiced within its walls*. Let every organ of the body be called by its right name,—as the arches or pillars of a building; the angles or triangles of geometrical figures; the petals or the stamens of flowers,—and the absurd notions that have driven a study so important to the preservation of life from the conversation and the teachings of home, disappear.

It is often said that "a little learning is a dangerous thing." This is untrue. In the practice of medicine it is found that even a little knowledge of the various branches of medical science is useful to the patient and to his attendant; that the observations he is capable of making greatly assist the physician; that his description of the symptoms is more reliable; that the physician's counsels are more strictly observed;

that the intercourse between physician and patient is more satisfactory. The fears of nervous people, which seem to have given rise to that saying, invariably spring from ignorance. Knowledge lessens fear, while it enhances vigilance and circumspection.

Delicacy is undoubtedly a charming characteristic of woman; nay, it is to her what perfume is to a flower; but true knowledge never trespasses upon delicacy. Ignorance leads to coarseness and slovenliness of thought, to insinuation and suspicion; and therein lies the vulgar fear of knowing anything regarding the human economy.

During a continued family medical practice of twenty years, it has fallen to the lot of the author to see many girls driven to invalidism by ignorance and neglect; also, many young married women who were quickly prostrated by the natural duty of bearing and rearing their children; even nursing seems to have become the business of the cow, rather than the contribution of the mother. This strange and almost fatal transference is not from the indifference of the mother towards performing a sacred duty to her child, but from her physical inability. The ratio of mortality of infants has thereby greatly increased, and yet there seems to be no remedy. The so-called "summer complaint," that mows down children like a scythe, is, in most instances, induced by this unnatural feeding of infants.

In the face of these startling facts, is it not the

physician's duty, nay, the parent's, to raise the young with a thorough knowledge of the laws of health? A diseased plant can produce but sickly shoots. To improve the physical condition of our race, we must begin with the young. The girls of to-day are the mothers of the future, and upon their health, more than upon that of the fathers, will depend the vigor and the strength of the generations to come. It is to them, therefore, that we dedicate this work; it is to them that we commend it, for, if they heed its suggestions, if they practice its precepts, although imperfect in construction and limited in extent, it will guide them safely through many a vicissitude that otherwise would plunge them into the afflictions, not only of a diseased body, but of diseased and feeble offspring hereafter.

This little volume is offered to the Mothers of the land, for their guidance and that of their Daughters; to teachers and guardians of young girls, for help in their difficult and delicate task; to young women, for their instruction in the most important interest of their lives. It is written as for my own daughter, and is inscribed to her; and when she is of the proper age to need and understand it, her mother will put it into her hands. With this object before me and the desire to benefit my kind, the following pages have been written.

T. S. V.

MOTHERS AND DAUGHTERS.

CHAPTER I.

THE MOTHER'S DUTY.

THIS little volume will be devoted to the physical perfection of woman; and in the effort to impart to her a knowledge without which her health must be in constant peril, the mother, and through her, the daughter, will be addressed in the relation they sustain towards each other; the mother as the wise and faithful counselor of the daughter, and the latter as the very inception of the coming mother; two halves which, united, complete the circle of woman's life, the unbroken ring of physical and moral continuity.

We feel no hesitation in addressing the mother, who, having passed through the vicissitudes of a girl's life and progressively risen into the mother's sphere, is conscious of the inadequate knowledge of the daughter; while it is far more difficult to address the girl, who, self-satisfied and in the delusion of the untaught, may not comprehend our solicitude. But if a girl can descend from the wings of sentimentality and see herself as a human being, having a physical nature, and subject to all its laws for good and for evil, this treatise may be of sufficient importance not only to claim her recognition, but to secure her gratitude.

A girl, who, like a morning rose-bud, enters into the first development of that life which will soon ripen into effulgent beauty, and disseminate around exquisite perfume, may too soon wither, like many others who have been treated inconsistently with the true principles of life and health.

It is hard for her, at the age when she sees life through a kaleidoscope that yields but beautiful and ever-changing colors, and dreams poetically of sentimental pictures, to come down to actual matter, and to the study of the laws that regulate it. Yet, should she make the attempt in earnest, she would soon find that there is as much of the wonderful and of the beautiful in this constitution of hers as there is in the exquisite flower that adorns her bosom.

It is sad to reflect upon the fact that that very knowledge of ourselves, so necessary to our preservation, is looked upon as the realm of grosser minds, and unworthy to be inquired into. It is still more sad, that parents, and mothers particularly, with a full understanding of its importance, through educational prejudices too frequently evade a branch of education so important to the well-being of their children. Prudery, mock and false modesty, have cast into early graves many young women who would otherwise have adorned society with their presence, and with love, virtue, prosperity and health aided in the great problem of human happiness.

It may be useless to attempt to discuss here, or determine, the causes that have thus deflected feminine education from the study of the human economy. Whatever they may be, the medical man is often brought in contact with the sad results of this illogical prudery. Many girls grow into womanhood only to perish as soon as they become mothers, in consequence of their ignorance of the simplest rules that would preserve their lives. A mother who sends her daughter from the paternal roof to become a wife, ignorant of the laws that will govern her as such, is guilty of a crime of omission which may consign that daughter to a life of misery.

Nature prepares a human being, as it does everything else, for the destiny designed for it; hence growth, as to time, size, shape, etc., is in conformity with the requirements of that specific object. Animals destined to but a limited sphere of action grow quickly, and are short-lived; animals whose sphere is greater, requiring a more refined intellect, and a more enduring muscular system, require longer time, and their growth is regulated by an unalterable method which cannot be improved, but may be damaged. If it is interesting to watch the growth of a plant, to study its physical life and to provide for its necessities so as to have it grow beautiful and yield abundantly, how much more so should it be to watch the growth of our children, to become intimately acquainted with their physical necessities in order to have them grow beautiful and luxuriant, and to yield abundantly?

Look at our girls, and particularly those of that class whose means are such as to enable them to leave the rough work of life for the education of their mental faculties, and from whom we should expect that knowledge which would make them thrive better than those of that less fortunate class whose life is a struggle of physical endurance. Are they healthier, stronger and more beautiful than their less favored sisters? No. What a commentary upon refined society! It is among the former that the scythe of death is busiest. What excuse have fathers and mothers, teachers and principals of educational institutions, for this criminal state of things? Is it that they are afraid to taint the minds of the young with prurient ideas? Can the knowledge of truth be injurious to the human mind? No knowledge, that will lead the mind, however young, to understand the work that impels it to continue an existence, can be injurious to it. "Forewarned, forearmed." That instruction will suggest the avoidance of those mistakes which imperil life, morally as well as physically. The knowledge of evil teaches how to avoid it; the knowledge of right teaches how to pursue it. Away, then, with false modesty in teaching what will preserve the health of the young, and what will enhance their moral development! The fear of knowledge belongs to the coward; and the fear of imparting knowledge is the mark of only such weak creatures, mentally, as cannot trust themselves, and to whom should not be entrusted the education of children.

Nevertheless, pulpits and educational chairs are full of such intellectual weakness.

The body is not corruption, uncleanliness, pollution: it is a grand conception; it is a marvelous work; it is beautiful. Its symmetry, its strength, its health, should be maintained. Body and mind cannot be separated; when that is done death ensues. No mind without a body; and what is a body without a mind? The mind cannot be improved at the expense of the body; their correlation is such that to do violence to one is to injure the other. A puny mind in a strong body is a monstrosity; a puny body with a strong mind is another. Their relations are mutual; both must be cultivated or both must perish. Then comes the corruption so constantly preached!

Woman, delicate and fragile from her very birth, is destined to become a mother, with all the sufferings and dangers attendant upon this exalted and beautiful privilege. She cannot therefore but excite the greatest interest, sympathy, and solicitude.

She has scarcely entered the charmed time of youth, and tasted the pleasures of life, ere she finds herself bound to periodical occurrences which demand her constant attention and the knowledge of her physical nature; for here is a process to which she is subject monthly, which, if disregarded, may imperil her health and even her life. From that moment, and for thirty years after, this demand will be made upon the system, requiring the utmost vigilance lest irregularities occur that reflect upon her general economy. Yet when one thinks of how many causes, some of which, even apparently trivial, can derange this process of nature, one shudders at the ignorance of our women regarding the means of preserving its integrity. And still more may we marvel at the indifference or neglect of the science that must acquaint girls with the physical laws of their existence, when we think of the consequences of such neglect; for out of a divergence from a periodical, normal continuance of that process, come such maladies as general weakness, neuralgias, spasms, hysteria, nervous headaches, backaches, which so disharmonize the whole system as to render the woman useless as a wife, feeble as a mother, worthless as a co-laborer, uninteresting as a friend, until, conscious of her own disability, and destined to pain and suffering, she feels that life is but a burden.

In the face of this our mothers and teachers are afraid or unwilling to instruct her!

Her very delicacy of construction should secure our greatest efforts for its preservation. In looking at a woman, young and beautiful, we would rather believe her a graceful flower on the meadow of life than a creature surrounded by all kinds of perils threatening her very existence. We need reflect but an instant upon the numerous vicissitudes to which she is destined, and the fact that her progress in life is through storms and dangers, to convince ourselves that her careeer should be assisted with all the knowledge and moral support we are able to give. Let not our admiration for her modesty lead us into the mistake that ignorance of her physical nature is the best means to secure the purity of her mind; for sooner or later she will herself find the rugged path and rightfully blame us for not forewarning her, and supplying her with the staff that would have enabled her to climb the rocks with safety, and overcome all the obstacles in her way.

Modesty is a trait that well becomes woman. It is attractive by its very reservations. It never satiates inquiry by complete revelation. It is pleasing, because its lights and shades are mellow, and are seen only through a haze of refining delicacy. Modesty adds to the beauty of character as pink adds to the beauty of the alabaster skin. But of modesty we discover two kinds: first, timid modesty, an offspring of ignorance, the shrinking of one who fears to tread upon unknown ground; then, a modesty true and self-reliant, possessed of the full knowledge of the dignity of womanhood. The modest girl should yet be learned in the demands of propriety, for her own well-being, and for her own and others' happiness.

Timid modesty may win friends, but not retain them; it may awaken curiosity, which shall grow into fervor and be mistaken for love. But, as ignorance ceases, in the same proportion timid modesty vanishes; and then, disenchanting truth comes forth in defiance of sentiment. Ignorance is not innocence. Dignified modesty, springing from self-respect and self-knowledge, stands invulnerable and unchangeable. A woman thus endowed will be dignified in her love, self-reliant and strong in her affections. Such modesty conquers man's love and respect, and holds him through all the trying experiences of married life. Knowledge, therefore, is no enemy to modesty; on the contrary, it enriches that lovely quality with the candor of truth, and a sense of rectitude which endears woman to all her associates.

There is nothing debasing in a study that teaches the anatomy and physiology of one's own mechanism; nothing prurient in the knowledge of the laws that govern it. It is through ignorance that these laws are violated, and that the precepts of virtue and the rules for health are disregarded.

We conjure then the mother, the natural protector of her offspring, to instruct her daughter in the multifarious changes to which she is liable, that the sufferings which might result therefrom be avoided.

Such instruction, coming, as it should, from the mother,

herself a woman who has passed through the various phases of life, will suggest and even secure on the part of the daughter the vigilance and discretion that will best protect her moral and physical life.

Convinced of the truth that girls suffer from an ignorance of the principal functions of their sex; convinced that mothers and teachers, through a mistaken sense of delicacy, and often through ignorance as well, are loth or unwilling to convey to a girl a knowledge so important to her well-being—not for the period of her girlhood only, but for the successive ones of womanhood and motherhood—we have devoted great care to the preparation of this volume, which, while it may instruct, will not excite morbid fancies, and in which the parent and the teacher will find a safe monitor on a subject of so much moment to the health of girls under their guidance. Ruskin says:

"Thus, then, you have first to mould her physical frame, and then, as the strength she gains will permit you, to fill and temper her mind with all knowledge and thoughts which tend to confirm its natural instincts of justice, and refine its natural tact of love.

. . . .

"The first of our duties to her—no thoughtful persons now doubt this—is to secure for her such physical training and exercise as may confirm her health and perfect her beauty; the highest refinement of that beauty being unattainable without splendor of activity and of delicate strength."

To the performance of this holy duty the author hopes

that those entrusted with the care and direction of the present generation of girls will find a helpful guide in this little volume, the result of conscientious study and long experience in family practice.

CHAPTER II.

A VEXED QUESTION.

ERE the topics of this volume are brought to the study of any girl she will probably have reached that age when she is willing to lay aside playthings for the soberer work of life. In her daily avocations and in the attainment of general knowledge she becomes aware that this world contains an immensity of things which will require all her industry, her deepest thoughts, her most earnest attention, to comprehend, to acquire, to estimate. As she in time becomes able to solve one problem after another, she will perceive that knowledge is obtained only through diligence and by a systematic, graduated method of study; that one step brings her nearer to another, until she attains an intellectual height that seemed at first beyond her reach. All undertakings of any magnitude appear difficult at first, and often deter the lazy or the weak of purpose from starting, appalled at obstacles that he has not yet examined; while the industrious and wise go, looking forward, hourly decreasing the distance between themselves and the object of their desire, rejoicing at progress, stimulating vigor with hope, until they finally reach the goal with a full sense of victory. The man of success does not stop there, for others are abreast of him; and he must win. His manhood, his ambition, his very success, spur him forward, until the laggard drops behind in the hopeless attempt at competition. This race for attainment is an attribute of civilized man, and its object is a noble one. Body and mind are engaged in the strife, and it would be but a vain attempt if these should perish in the endeavor.

And this brings us directly to our subject—one often neglected; one which never leaves you in life, if in death; neither in joy, nor in sorrow, in sickness, nor in health; it is your best friend, or your worst enemy; one that you should know and control. Imagine an object upon which so much of your welfare depends, and then say if you would not shield it against every accidental evil? Would you not study it, that you might best serve and protect it? What then can it be—this object of such transcendent importance? It is *your own body!* Let not the reader hesitate to descend to a subject so unworthy, so unpoetical. Be assured that poetry, art and philosophy have failed to produce so grand, so perfect, so beautiful an object as the human body; that science and art, philosophy and poetry, are never more attractive than when they treat of that very object which so many affect to despise.

You have probably been on board a steamship and visited the engine-room; if not, go at your earliest opportunity. Notice those huge shining arms of steel, which, although inanimate, pull and push with the power of a thousand horses; notice those wheels with interlocking teeth, revolving with a power that would lift a thousand tons! You are amazed, and wonder what would happen if one should snap. You wonder, also, what power impels those blocks of iron to act as if life were in them, and whence the power comes. Descend still deeper into the vessel, and you will come to heated furnaces, and find men engaged in feeding them with tons of coal. There is the motive power; it is in that black coal. It wants but a spark of fire, and some oxygen from the air, to convert its mass into heat; heat to convert the water into steam; steam to expand and lift the pistons that set the whole machinery in motion. Singly, the iron, the coal, the oxygen, would be inert; brought together, they need but a spark of fire to develop this wondrous power. That little spark of fire, then, is the initiative force of an energy that drives four thousand tons of matter through the waves of the ocean at the rate of twenty miles an hour. You ponder this exhibition of power, and admire the ingenuity of man, who taught himself to adapt mechanism to force, and force to mechanism, in a manner to produce such astonishing results. Your enthusiasm strengthens your courage, and you hope that you too will in time add your atom of intellect and ingenuity to this great capacity of your kind. Yet, that marvelous conception that you have witnessed is the resultant work of the brains and hands of millions of men, who in successive generations have only added and added, each something, to the other's labor, and together they obtain this grand achievement.

But there is a machine of much more wonderful construction and power, the conception of which is of but one mind. A machine, automatic, self-feeding, and self-preserving; whose motive-power was a "fiat" (the first spark); a beginning which has baffled all the investigations of the philosophers; a beginning which, not being explainable, must be a faith. This machine, so perfect in all its details, so marvelous in its adaptation, so beautiful in its execution, is—*yourself*. Need you go to the steamship to be surprised? Need you look at her engine to detect intellectual power? No; look at your hand, at a hair from your head, and you will find enough to admire, to reflect upon, and, in its Cause, to love, to worship. Yet that hand, that hair, lie before you at all times, and go unnoticed.

All that art and science have devised and accomplished since the beginning of the world is but a trifle in comparison with the works of nature. Moreover, man, however intellectual, cannot create; he can only adapt that which is already created; avail himself of nature's laws, of nature's deeds, to model, to imitate, to construct, to apply what may be of benefit to himself.

In this study we shall take man as our subject; nay, the best part of him,—Woman; and in the most beautiful and critical era of her existence,—Maidenhood. In this connection, we will apply the term "girlhood," or "maidenhood," to that period in a young woman's life when, for the first time, her system assumes the functions peculiar to her sex.

Timidly she now turns into this path, for hereafter she will be widely separated from the boy companions of her childhood, with whom she has had everything in common. Physical necessity will cause her to glide farther and farther away from them, and her mental and physical culture will prepare her henceforth for a life utterly different from theirs.

A story is told of Achilles, when in hiding from his enemies, that to discover him among the maidens with whom he was playing, dressed in their own costume, the stratagem of exhibiting jewels and arms was resorted to. Nature spoke; the girls rushed to the jewels, and Achilles to the arms. In proportion to growth, the boy loses all taste for effeminate things, while the girl still cultivates it, and even with a higher degree of appreciation and refinement.

Physically, the difference becomes no less striking. The boy's rounded limbs yield their fat, and assume the irregularities of the knotty, powerful muscle; his arms now lift weights that his whilom fair companion can hardly move; his legs carry him over mountains and over plains where she cannot follow. But, while nature seems engaged in giving the boy strength, she is assiduously laboring to give the girl beauty; and as an author has said: "The beautiful face of a woman seems to be the most finished work of creation."

Here they part as girl and boy, to meet as man and woman; and when they meet again, the change is so great that one scarcely recognizes the other. The recollection of the past brings them no nearer; had they parted as man and woman in intimate relations, they would now meet with the full recognition of each other's claim; but the boy left a girl and now meets a woman; the girl parted from a boy and now meets a man. They were friends of old; but they find that they must actually make one another's acquaintance, as if they were strangers.

In this separation, the moral is no less striking and peculiar than the physical change. The man now looks upon the woman as a weaker being whom he is bound to protect. He manifests his interest by many acts that refined society calls gallantry. Woman generally acquiesces, even with a sense of gratified vanity, in this position. Such relation gradually becomes intensified, until the man assumes control of the woman. It is this that has caused so much dispute, and excited more comment and passionate discussion amongst philosophers and moralists, philanthropists and romancists than almost any other question. Still, their rhapsodies and harangues have accomplished but little; and man still lends his strong arm to the willing receiver, who rarely considers it a burden, although wiseacres will insist that it is only an imposition upon her.

The reason for man's general advantage in power is a very simple if not a very lofty one. In a word, it lies in his physical superiority and efficiency.

In the struggle for existence, health and strength are the shields for self-preservation—the weapons for the battle. No one, however rich, however exalted, can avoid that struggle; and here it is that man is superior, naturally taking the lead in the government and the domination of the world. In certain historical periods, when men gave themselves up to effeminate habits, they ceased to be powerful, and were conquered and overwhelmed by nations of men who had cultivated energy, maintained mental and physical activity, and economized vital force by proper restraint upon the passions and the vanities of social life.

In the race of life the strongest wins; and that there is a constant and continuous struggle among all animals, man included, for supremacy, is incontestable; equally incontestable is it, that the healthier and stronger the individual, the greater is the chance for success. The healthiest and the strongest is even the preferred, for health and strength is beauty. Among the lower orders of the animal kingdom the battle for life is fiercest, and often the weak has to die that the strong may live. With humanity, the battle of life is not always a matter of physical strength, for the highly developed mind controls action; and action, thus controlled, is superior to mere brute force. But great conceptions, resulting in concentration and organization of power, are the work of healthy minds. Hence, body and mind, "pari passu," act in the strife for self-protection, and *health* is the essence of the strength that conquers.

It is a common grievance that man has a better chance than woman in this struggle; that he has arrogated the power to govern both sexes; that he has made woman subservient, and driven her from law and government, of which she is, nevertheless, a subject. We will not deny the assertion, but we will indicate the reason by an example of its action.

The United States government employs in the various Departments at the capital many hundreds of women, and Congress has provided that, in the clerical force, no distinction shall be made except on account of fitness. If the women do not rise in office in the same proportion as the men, it is not the fault of the law, or the arrogance of the men; nor is it on account of mental, but of physical, disability. Scores of women daily leave the Departments exhausted, overcome by nervousness or by ailments peculiar to their sex. Were they healthy and strong, they would rival men, with the chances in their favor; for it is admitted that they excel in sobriety, industry, carefulness and diligence. As it is in those offices, so it is in every department of life.

The advantage of man is in his training and education and consequent strength; his physical existence is not dwarfed by stringent regulations of mistaken propriety to take him from the fields of play and exercise; his body is allowed to grow untrammeled by tight lacing, not deformed by unphysiological vestment, not exposed by partial covering. His limbs are free to run, leap or wrestle; his chest is clear, and he grows as nature provided that all animals should grow—strong, robust and self-reliant.

So should woman grow, and then her struggle for existence would gain such proportions as to compel the present stronger sex to acknowledge her, not only as his equal, but as his ally in all the great undertakings of life.

In the order of creation man and woman are only the complement of each other; and one has but to study the law of adaptation to discover that, in the fitness of things, they are in perfect harmony. They act two distinctive parts, but in a co-ordinate manner, so that they are auxiliary, rather than subordinate, to each other—imperfect in separation, perfect in union. It cannot be attempted, therefore, to make woman identical with man, but to make her perfect in her sphere, and by true development of natural capacities enable her to perform the work adapted to her organization. That is the true equality to be demanded for the two sexes—a chance for *equality in excellence*, whatever the respective vocation or adaptation may be.

Sterne, in one of his sermons, says: "Had God intended to make woman the master of man, He would have drawn her from his head; had He intended to make her his slave, He would have drawn her from his feet; but drawing her from his side He made her his companion and his equal."

However, it is not the purpose of this book to discuss social questions, except so far as they concern the health of our girls and, through them, of mankind; and particularly is it not its intent to discuss the social equality claimed by some of the more advanced adherents of "woman's rights" (vulgarly so-called), a "cause" which has perhaps created more commotion than progress towards the welfare of woman.

The world seems to have settled that man, as the representative of physical force and physical endurance, should be pre-eminent in the control of human affairs. Not that intellect, in which woman might claim equality, if not pre-eminence, has been deemed secondary or subordinate to physical power; but because physical power is in fact the exponent of the intellect, the *executive officer* of all mental operations. As man possessed both physical and mental strength, there would be no alternative but to accept him as the leader.

It is from the self-evident quality of these truths that we are forced to feel the essential difference existing between the sexes, manifesting itself even at a very tender age, and which, in due course, becomes thoroughly defined when they assume the parts in the plan of creation imposed by their respective conditions.

But, at the same time, the very ease with which man instinctively takes and woman unthinkingly yields the larger share of employment, of emolument, of influence, authority and power, is an enforcement of the lesson that this book is meant to teach—that bodily vigor is

A VEXED QUESTION. 25

the foundation of success in life. And whether it be in the various avenues of trade and professional life, or in that richer and happier realm, the family, from which woman's influence has its broadest and grandest sweep, the rule still holds. "A sound mind *in a sound body*" is that which alone will give woman her true place in nature and in society.

CHAPTER III.

PHYSIOLOGY AS A MORAL TEACHER.

OF all laws of nature none are so important to humanity as the laws of health, for, as we have seen, without health man can accomplish but little.

Health is that condition of the body in which all its organs and tissues perform their functions without interruption; any other would be disease. It behooves us, then, to understand those functions, lest we unwittingly interfere with their free and normal operations.

Woman's organization is more complex than man's, hence she should be a greater student of her nature than even man should be of his. The finer and more complicated the machinery, the more profound the study necessary, is a dictum which we cannot gainsay. It devolves, then, upon woman to earnestly and profoundly consider all the operations of the organs special to her sex.

There are narrow-minded people who do not recognize this necessity; for in life or in death, in the normal or the abnormal, in the act or the accident, they declare, one should see but the finger of God—the exhibition of his will. They are so well acquainted with the will of the Almighty that they do not think it temerity to thus pronouce his judgment. Were their assumptions true, the very word *accident* should be expunged from the vocabulary of every idiom, as an accident could not be an accident if preordained by any power. Believers in

God should rather be terrified at the idea of holding him responsible for their infractions of his laws. The laws are ordained and enacted, and all matter, organic or inorganic, is made subservient to them; and neither the most moral nor the most wicked, the most learned nor the most ignorant, can change them. The existence of these laws should, then, be the signal-light of our actions, which should be watched with eager solicitude; for, if we sleep in our bunk when the beacon-light is in view, and then awake to find ourselves stranded upon the shore, helpless and bleeding, would it not be illogical to prostrate ourselves before the Almighty and thank him for his visitation? What a plausible argument for the captain of a ship, who, having abandoned the helm for his bed in the moment of danger, would plead that the Almighty lulled him asleep that the wicked passengers might be punished for their sins! The narrow-minded man who affects to believe that every motion, however accidental, is decreed then and there by the will of God, would probably be the first to visit the captain with his indignation, and vote to hang him to the mast.

An accident is always the result of the violation of a natural law, whether such violation has occurred through ignorance or ill-will; and human responsibility is just in proportion to the knowledge of such law. When the law is written or expounded there can be no just plea for our ignorance; and it would be insane, if not wicked, to hold the law-maker responsible for our infringement. God, unlike Caligula, has not placed his laws at such a height that human vision cannot reach them. Even animals, without reason, instinctively act in obedience to the laws of nature, self-preservation being the motive that impels them. The bird takes its flight southward at the approach of winter; the dog selects the grass that is medicine to its system; the horse pricks up its ears and listens at the approach of danger. Man has more than instinct—he has reason. His reasoning powers lead him to comparison; comparison yields a knowledge that is accumulative; his knowledge he can impart to others, which is education, and to which every every human being can add his bounty of experience.

Typhoid fever appears in the midst of a family and carries to an untimely grave the young and the strong. This is startling! But a sanitary engineer comes to investigate the cause, finds a pool of stagnant water giving rise to a deadly effluvium; the pool is drained, the cause removed, and the people residing thereabout are no longer attacked by the fatal malady.

Smallpox appears in a community; in a short time a mantle of terror spreads over all its members. A scientific hygienist, acquainted with the laws of propagation by contagion, isolates the unfortunate ones afflicted with the disease, destroys or disinfects everything that may convey the virus; the disease is arrested and the community saved.

The plague visits a badly built and overcrowded city, London, and carries away one hundred thousand inhabitants in a terribly short space of time; the London fire occurs and burns down hundreds of acres of miserably ventilated and dirty dwellings; the city is rebuilt on hygienic principles, ventilation and drainage are regarded, overcrowding forbidden, and the plague appears not again, although hundreds of years elapse.

What miserable helplessness, if people should fold their arms in the face of danger and wait for the decree of Providence to free them from the scourge! That they would be punished for their cowardly inertness there is no doubt, but the punishment would be self-administered.

The study of cause and effect has corrected a thousand evils, and will go on correcting them so long as, in the consciousness of sacred duty, man has regard for the laws of nature and obeys them. Where knowledge is attainable it is criminal to avoid it. The ignorance of the laws of health, which learned men have placed before the people, is a deflection from moral duty, the fruit of which must be illness of the body, and destruction of life. Laws, human or divine, are made for the welfare of all, and it is presumption to suppose that they might be suspended in a particular case simply because the offender regrets the infraction, and invokes the Great Power to make him an exception. The prayer of the infractionist is but hypocrisy; for the law must take its course, and not be suspended that a criminal may clear his conscience. Sincere repentance appeals to human sympathy, as well as to divine; but while the reward for his repentance may be a future happiness, in this or in the other world, he must now expiate the penalty for his present crime.

This digression, *quasi* theological, may be deemed an intrusion, introduced on the false plea of physical education; but, indifference to the study of the physical laws that govern our economy is so general and so flagrant, encouraged even by professors of religion, that we are driven to trespass upon a dominion we would rather avoid, that nothing may remain unobserved that has any bearing upon the physical welfare of our fellow-men.

If that anxiety has driven us beyond the sphere of a medical teacher let it be our apology.

CHAPTER IV.

MORAL AND PHYSICAL CHARACTERISTICS OF WOMAN.

THE external appearance of an animal does not always indicate its sex. The peculiarities that characterize each sex rarely become pronounced before childhood passes into youth. Boys are often mistaken for girls and girls for boys at that early age when it is not thought necessary to dress them in garments distinctive of their sex. It is later, when nature prepares each one for its ultimate physical destiny, that the traits peculiar to each respective sex become plainly manifested. At that point of time the two sexes commence to vary in their mode of growth, and continue to do so until the full and mature size of man and woman is attained.

This mode of growth, so different from that of childhood, is not only made apparent by the difference of form and shape of the body, but also by the manifestation of the mind in the development of intellectual power, of the passions, the normal dispositions, and the æsthetics of social and refined life. As man departs from childhood he acquires courage, energy, and all the qualities that lead to the strife for conquest, for honor, or for gain. Woman, on the other hand, cultivates the nobler passions of the heart that direct her to devotion, to charity and to love. Man's physical development is consonant with his moral inclination, and gives him the nervous force, the muscular strength, to achieve the plans of his conception. The childlike roundness of his limbs, the smoothness and complexion of his skin, gradually disappear, to be replaced by the irregularities of developed muscles, by deeper and ruddier shades of color, by stronger and deeper voice. The timidity of his youth is changed into a courage that knows no fear; he is stronger in contention than in peace. His height is increased beyond that of woman; his carriage is firm and decided; all his pursuits indicate force. Such characteristics are manly, and are recognized even by the parents as the heralds of power and success.

Woman, physically, is comparatively weaker, but her nervous system is more impressionable, and is, therefore, more prone to change. Being impressible, she detects good or evil with quickness, and responds to her impressions with energy. She repels an odious object without hesitation; she embraces a pleasing one with enthusiasm. This sensibility plays an important *rôle* in the conventional life of humanity; it denounces dishonor; it repels injustice; it rewards merit and virtue, and it animates charity. Her tenderness conquers positiveness, her affection overpowers even reason.

As a result of her natural traits and peculiarities of culture she is distinguished for her love of humanity, often manifested in her compassion for sufferers, in her charity for the needy, in the conciliations brought about through her mediatorship. Her mission being one of peace, of charity and love, she is an easement to the rugged life of man; a refreshment to his heated brain; a rest to his forcing, contriving, swaying, dominating spirit. "She orders with a caress, she threatens with a tear; her empire is goodness."—(Rousseau.)

The poets have sung pæans in her honor; muses have been invoked in her praise.

The brute bravery of man is in her contrasted by a moral courage that has no bounds. Her immolation on the altar of love and virtue reaches beyond the capacity of man. The history of revolutions, wars and famines has given striking illustrations of this power of self-sacrifice. Her prowess is seldom induced by ambition, by pretension, or by lower passions. Her love is the motive power of her moral greatness. She abounds in patriotism; she defies a giant in the defense of her little ones. Man unfurls the banner of freedom, and in the storm of battle he is foremost in the charge of the braves. Woman voluntarily moulders in the dungeon or the bastile by the side of her father or husband, that he may not perish alone, or live uncared for; with him she shares the gallows or the guillotine. This timid creature, who would tremble at the sight of an insect, will scale a prison or a fortress, open her breast to a dagger, unflinchingly stand before a tiger, lend her bosom to the dying Roman, suffer cold, hunger, and death that the one she loves may be saved, or the principle she maintains may be vindicated.

During the French revolution, which for terror, blind passion and incarnate deviltry has hardly had its parallel in the history of the world, woman played a conspicuous part; where she hated her ferocity was unbounded; where she loved, her love was divine.

The following pertinent story is told of Mlle. de Sombreuil: Her father was condemned to perish under the guillotine, where in the previous twenty-four hours hundreds had been decapitated. Mlle. de Sombreuil asked the price of her father's deliverance. The cruel answer was that she should drink a goblet of human blood. The condition was so inhuman that these murderers thought it beyond even the devotion of this martyr. She who, under ordinary circumstances, would have fainted at a drop of blood, took the chalice thus contemptuously offered, and drank the sickening draught. She dropped into convulsions immediately afterwards, this being, of course, induced by the great mental effort to conquer her horror and disgust at the libation. Her father's life was thus saved, but only to be spent in a dungeon: she did not leave him then; but there in a dark cell of the Bastile, she shared his imprisonment until the reign of terror ceased and humanity prevailed. All her fellow prisoners shed tears at the exhibition of such filial love, at a time when the satanic passions seemed to have been unchained amidst that benighted people.

But it was for Mme. de Rosambo to make even grander this greatest of virtues. In perceiving Mlle. de Sombreuil, Mme. de Rosambo exclaimed: "You have had the glory of saving your father; I shall have the consolation of dying with mine."

Such is woman! Volumes have been written, and many more could be compiled, with instances of this self-immolation of woman on the altar of love, virtue, piety and devotion. But as it is not our purpose to write the romance of woman's mental and moral life, we must pass on to our intention of examining more immediately into her physical life and development.

From the time when the difference arises in the development of the boy and the girl, the former in a short time loses all his primitive appearance, whereas woman perfects her already beautiful lines of contour. From this time her growth is more rapid than his; both anatomists and physiologists concur in the statement that this growth is physical as well as moral, and that the summit of woman's growth is attained at the age of twenty-one, while that of man is put at twenty-five. Legislators, recognizing this difference, have decreed that her majority shall be at eighteen, while that of the man is decreed at twenty-one, or in proportion to this established theory of growth. Herr Teufelsdröckh's hard philosophy recognized this difference when he said, "I have heard affirmed, surely in jest, by not unphilanthropic persons, that it were a real increase of human happiness could all young men from the age of nineteen be covered under barrels, or rendered otherwise invisible, and there left to follow their lawful studies and callings till they emerged, sadder and wiser, at the age of twenty-five. With which suggestion, at least as considered in the light of a practical scheme, I need scarcely say that I in no wise coincide. Nevertheless it is plausibly urged that as young ladies are, to mankind, precisely the most delightful in those years, so young gentlemen do then attain their maximum of detestability. Such gawks are they, and foolish peacocks, and yet with such a vulturous hunger for self-indulgence, so obstinate, obstreperous, vain glorious; in all senses so froward and so forward." (Carlyle's "Sartor Resartus.")

The nubile girl of eighteen treats her contemporary of the opposite sex with more condescension than deference; more patronizingly than would be becoming towards an equal. But he is not her equal; she has risen to the dignity of womanhood; he is still distant from the realm of his manhood. This advantage in her youth she loses, however, in more advanced life; for while he is still in the ripe season of his manhood, she has passed into maturity, after which vitality declines.

The time and scale of growth, as already stated, is thus shown to have relation to the law of necessary continuation of force, or of mental and physical capacity.

In height and volume the two sexes differ; woman never attaining the stature of man, the average of her stature being one-sixth less than his. In her dimensions, and the relation of her organs, the following difference is also apparent. Transversely separated in halves, man's line of division would be at the separation of the lower limbs, while the line in woman would be higher. The shortness of her limbs is in part compensated for by greater length of neck and body, which induces a graceful undulation of movement in her walk. While nature has provided her with dimensions and forms adapted to the necessity of maternity, with room for the reception and indwelling of a rapidly growing guest, it has not neglected the attributes of symmetry and elegance.

The breasts, which in man remain in a rudimentary condition, in woman develop, become elevated, and marked by roundness of contour, fineness of texture and delicacy of color. These organs, so wonderfully organized for the preparation and provision of the nourishment of her infant, give also added grace and elegance to woman's form.

Her lower limbs are larger, rounder, and softer than man's. They are further apart, from the hips to the knees, and approach nearer together from the knee to the foot, than in man. The direction of her limbs corresponds to her wider basin, and is in harmony with the laws of equilibrium. This conformation manifestly expresses the preparations of nature for gestation and child-bearing.

The foot and hand are smaller, plumper and more delicate, and give a finish to an already beautiful body.

Her bones are smaller, lighter and whiter; their processes less acute and less pronounced, more spongy, oily, and supple in organization. Her pelvis, or basin, is to be excepted from the above rule, for the side bones (innominata) are wider, and more oval than man's, giving to the lower trunk more breadth—a characteristic the uses of which we shall examine hereafter.

The muscles attain a greater development and stand out in bolder relief in man. His large and superficial ones can be traced through their whole course, even from above the surface of the skin. The external unevenness in man's muscles is partly due to the absorption of adipose tissue, which is generally found in abundance around the muscle of woman at all ages, and of man only in early youth; but, more particularly, to the greater development of each muscular fiber, from the greater exercise that man gives to it in his plays, his games, and his general habits. A muscle is a bundle of such fibers, larger in the centre than at each extremity. The number of fibers composing a certain muscle in man need not be greater than that composing the same muscle in woman; but, having attained a greater volume from the exercise above described, the muscle is proportionately larger, and marked by those elevations and that firmness recognized as manifestations of better development. This uneven and knotty appearance evinces strength and power.

The construction and functions of the muscles are the same in both sexes. The muscles of woman's face, however, respond more promptly to the emotions of her mind, which may be owing to her comparative powerlessness in controlling mental impression. The muscles of her face being, also, less salient than those of man, lend her an attractive expression of sweetness and benevolence. Her skin is more delicate and finer, more susceptible to the influence of air, or whatever object comes in contact with it. It is of a finer grain—the capillary vessels entering it very freely—and of such whiteness that the blue of her veins is seen through the transparency of the tissue. The complexion of her skin is generally lighter than that of man, and rarely is its white and velvety surface protected with hair.

The conformation of the chest of the two sexes is quite different; the man's lung is more conical, the apex being larger in woman, the base in man. Thus, while the chest of man grows broader downwards, in woman it is more elevated above, giving it the appearance of being fuller, while its contraction below is gradual and graceful. Comparatively, her lungs are smaller and lie higher, a conformation tending to give her more abdominal room for organs which man does not possess. But while the lung of woman is smaller, it is more active, thus making up in energy what is lost in volume. The arch of her ribs, also, is more acute, so that at every inspiration her chest rises higher than that of man; and this fact is very noticeable in woman particularly when she is under strong emotion. The heart follows the same principle of organization; for, while it is smaller in woman it beats quicker, thus, like the lungs, equilibrating the want of size by increase of energy.

The digestive apparatus is also organized with the same view to a free and roomy abdominal cavity. The stomach is longer but smaller, the liver less voluminous, and the intestines shorter in proportion.

There is nothing more beautiful in anatomy and physiology than this adaptation in the organization of the body. It seems that nature had a reason for every change, every curve, every prominence; and it is so not only in the human frame but throughout creation, whether animate or inanimate.

The voice, that mirror of the soul, is strikingly different in the two sexes; being more flexible and of sweeter tone in woman. This flexibility of the vocal organs, as well as of all the muscles of her throat, enables woman to cultivate music with more facility. More women sing than men. In the acquirement of languages woman is an easy adept, while man struggles to imitate sounds he can scarcely ever produce.

We have thus given some general points of difference found in the two sexes; but the principal features which eminently distinguish woman from man are of course the organs which adapt her to perform the holy and responsible functions of maternity. The consideration of these we shall now enter upon, under a deep sense of the importance, the delicacy, and the vital interest of the subject, trusting that these conscientious observations of an experienced physician, who writes as for his own wife and daughter, may be of real service to the mothers and daughters of our land.

CHAPTER V.

THE PELVIS,

AND ITS RELATION TO WOMAN'S SAFETY.

THE Pelvis is an important part of the skeleton in the study of the distinctive organs of woman. It is the bony basin, the outer edges of which form the hips, and which is spread out to uphold and support all the most important interior organs of the body. Behind, it commences at the lowest lumbar vertebra, that is, at the small of the back, and continues downwards to the end of the spine. Laterally, the hip-bones form its prominent parts, the sides of the basin sloping downwardly and inwardly, below the upper head of the thigh-bones. This would form a cone with its base upwards if it were closed in by bony structure in front, as it is on its sides and back. In front, however, the sides of the pelvis are open at the top, and coming down to meet each other are joined atthe lower extremity by two triangular arms, forming the pubis. Anatomically, all these bony parts are separate, each bearing a distinct name, such as "the Sacrum," behind, "Ossa Innominata," at the sides, and "Os Pubis," in front. The bones at the bottom of the pelvic basin, on which the body rests when in sitting posture, are called "Ischii."

All the above named bones knit together constitute one firm body, called *pelvis*, or *basin*. The cavity within this basin is not regular or straight, being somewhat bent and constricted in the middle like an old-fashioned barber's basin.

This constriction divides the cavity into two sections; the upper one being called by anatomists the "greater," and the lower one the "lesser," or the "*superior*" and "*inferior, straits.*"

The walls of the abdomen close and complete the cavity in front.

So far, this cavity has been spoken of as a distinct one, but in reality it is only a portion of the abdominal cavity, which reaches upward to the arch of the diaphragm at the base of the lungs. This great abdominal cavity, including that of the pelvis, contains above and on the right, the liver; in the center and at the lower extremity of the breast bone, the stomach; the spleen on the left; the kidneys behind, or about at the small of the back; the intestines filling up the largest portion of the cavity in the center, and the bladder and the rectum lying at the lowest end of the funnel-shaped space.

In woman, however, the womb occupies a space an inch or two below the navel, behind the small intestines and in front of the rectum. It lies about six inches above the entrance of the vagina, with which it connects, just as the small end of a pear (which is about the shape of the womb) would enter into a tube larger than its neck, but smaller than its body. In continuation with the upper end of the womb are the "Fallopian tubes" and the "ovaries," (the uses of which will be explained hereafter) which extend to the right and to the left, like the spread wings of a bat. The "ovaries" lie in the hollow on each side of the abdomen, formed by the projection of the hip-bones, about two inches below the crest. All these various organs are held in position in the abdominal cavity by a membrane called the "Peritoneum;" besides all these, there are arteries, veins, nerves, lymphatics, &c.

The pelvis is somewhat different in the two sexes, for very pertinent reasons. As a whole, the pelvis in the male is smaller but deeper; the bones are thicker. There are other, minor, differences in the construction and the diameters, but they would be of little interest or importance to the reader.

The two lower limbs are attached to the sides of the bony circle formed by the pelvis, and support, in the erect posture, all the weight of the upper part of the body.

Another important function of the pelvis is to enclose and protect the generative and digestive organs. During gestation, it sustains and gives a proper direction to the womb; and in labor it affords a safe passage to the child.

From this description, is evident the necessity to woman of perfection in the construction of the pelvis, who is to give birth to the child.

Since the pelvis has important relation to childbearing, it follows that in early life great care should be exercised that proper proportions may be secured, and deviations from normal conditions obviated. Its cavities and outlets are regarded by the physician with great interest, for upon them depends, in a great measure, the safety of the mother at delivery. Like all other bony structures, its development is gradual until the age of eighteen, and even later, when ossification seems to have reached its degree of perfection. During all these years of growth, the various bones of the pelvis are held together by muscular attachments, and by cartilaginous articulations. During the tender age of a girl, a fall, or badly applied vestments, causing pressure on any part of it, may disturb the normal position of the respective bones, and produce a distorted pelvis. Such an unfortunate occurrence might prove a serious malformation, that would impede the natural progress of labor.

At birth, the pelvis is extremely narrow and elongated, and of such inconceivably small dimensions that its cavity cannot contain several of the organs afterwards found in it; from which circumstance the protuberance of the abdomen, observed in the fœtus and in children at term, in great measure results. It is stated by anatomists, however, that its form changes by degrees as little girls advance in age; thus it is that the diameter from front to back, which measures two and seven-eighths (2 7-8) inches at nine years, will gradually increase until at the eighteenth year it will have acquired a length of four inches; while the transverse diameter, which at nine years of age is found to be about three inches, at eighteen years is four and one-half (4 1-2) inches.

It is not enough to bear in mind the general form or construction of the pelvis as already given; its mode of development should also claim attention. As the pelvis is not a single bone completed at birth, but, on the contrary, a system of bones whose union is accomplished only in years after birth, it devolves upon us to know its manner of growth, that it may not be exposed to accidents, to distortions, or to deviations.

We find that at birth and for several years after, the pelvis is divided into separate parts, each part being kept in juxtaposition to the others by elastic, fibrous ligaments and cartilages. There are no less than six such parts thus united, three on each side, having five distinct articulations or joints. It is true that these articulations do not allow as much freedom of motion as those of the elbows, knees, or other bony surfaces of the skeleton; but they are nevertheless movable, sliding one on the other and easily bent by compression, particularly during the tender period preceding puberty, and more or less, also, until the age of eighteen, when ossification has firmly secured the several parts together.

Mothers acquainted with these facts could not fail to appreciate our solicitude regarding the normal growth of this part of the body of woman. The tender care of the mother should therefore commence immediately after the birth of a girl. At this time it is usual for the nurse, for the sake of neatness, to apply a napkin to the child; but this napkin is often a cumbrous affair, badly adjusted. It is generally folded in a triangular form, the longest side drawn over the hips around the back and pinned in front of the abdomen. We have already stated that at this time of life the little pelvis is so incompletely developed, that the womb of a girl is out of its cavity and the protection of its bones. If that napkin is coarse and heavy, clumsily applied, or too tight around the abdomen, it may be that undue pressure is exerted over the prominence of the abdomen, thus causing the womb to descend, and induce, even at this early age, a displacement of that organ, which in turn may press upon the bladder, disabling the child from holding its water for a longer period than an hour. The frequent micturitions of infant girls may be due partly to this unsuspected pressure.

It is known, moreover, that at the tender age of infancy, the bones do not contain enough earthy matter to render them hard, and consequently they are pliable and easily bent. The broad bones of the pelvis are oblique; hence, constriction around the body may cause them to bend, thus changing the direction of growth, so that, instead of growing outwardly, they may be made to grow inwardly, restricting the development of the cavity to its minimum, instead of encouraging its width to the maximum.

In consideration of the above, the attendants should see that the bands and napkins applied to infants be so loose as to make *no pressure whatever*. Allowing a napkin to be a necessity for cleanliness, and even for decency, let it be pinned to the undershirt, or to a loose belt held in position by suspenders.

This freedom, so much recommended for the proper development of the pelvis, is not to be neglected even later, when girls attain the age which ushers them into society that awakens in the mind a desire for beauty of form, of manner, and of dress, for then they improperly lace their waists, carry weight upon their hips, and in various ways compress the surface and circumference of the pelvis.

When treating the subject of dress in other parts of this book, we shall enter more fully into a description of the ills attendant upon improper modes of dressing.

CHAPTER VI.

THE WOMB.

IN his work on *Maternity*, a book prepared for the guidance of young married women, the author has given a limited description of the womb and its appendages. Were it not that he conscientiously feels that even the younger woman ought to be acquainted with an organization peculiar to her sex, he would abstain from further description of the specifically female organs. It would be difficult for her to fully distinguish the unnatural from the true functions of those organs, without some knowledge of their peculiar construction and relations. From the moment that the girl becomes the woman, her moral and physical life becomes dependent upon a regular, unobstructed action of these organs; and it would seem that too much could not be said to enable her to foresee or prevent accidents, and to maintain the integrity of their relations.

The womb, in its original state, is a pear-shaped body, flattened before and behind, situated in the cavity of the pelvis, between the upper part of the bladder and the rectum. It is retained in its position by round and broad ligaments on each side, and projects downward into the upper end of the vagina. It lies obliquely, its upper end, or base, being directed upwards and forwards; its lower end, or apex, downwards and backwards, in the line with the *in*let of the pelvis, forming an angle with the vagina, the downward and forward direction of which corresponds to the cavity and *out*let of the pelvis.

The uterus or womb measures about three inches in length, two in breadth at its upper part, and an inch in thickness, and weighs from an ounce to an ounce and a half.

This pear-shaped body, for the sake of convenience, is by anatomists divided into two parts, the upper of which, called the *body*, is the largest, and comprises more than one-half the total length; the other, or lower portion, styled the *neck*, is smaller; a slight circular constriction serves to indicate externally the point of union of the body with the neck.

Essentially, the womb is a thick, powerful, and elastic muscle, which can become so expanded as to be as thin as a sheet of paper. During pregnancy it increases in size and weight, and becomes so dilated as to enclose within its cavity a child weighing twelve pounds or more, an after-birth (the spongy tissue which connects the child in the womb with its mother) weighing three or four pounds, and a pint or more of water. Its power of contractility also is so great, that during the process of labor it can expel all of the contents mentioned above, and reduce itself to a size very little beyond its original one before pregnancy.

Its cavity is lined by a thin, smooth and closely adherent mucous membrane, which continues through the fallopian tubes, and through its mouth connects with the mucous lining of the vagina.

The cavity of the uterus in its unoccupied condition is small in comparison with the size of the organ. If cut in two, from side to side, its cavity would represent a triangular fissure, two angles of which would be in continuation with the fallopian tubes at each side of the upper end of the uterus, and one with its mouth at the lower end. In the state of vacuity it could hardly be said that the womb contains a cavity, for the uterine walls are in contact throughout their extent, and hardly show more than a line of separation.

The form, size, and situation of the uterus vary at different periods of life and condition. At birth, it lies higher in the cavity of the abdomen, and its neck is considerably larger than its body. At puberty, it has attained the shape and proportions above described. During and after menstruation, the organ is enlarged and more vascular. During pregnancy, it increases in weight from one pound and a half to three pounds. After child-birth it nearly regains its usual size, weighing from two to three ounces, its cavity, however, remaining larger than in the former state. In old age it becomes shrunken, paler, and denser in texture.

CHAPTER VII.

FALLOPIAN TUBES AND OVARIES.

THE fallopian tubes are named from Fallopius, an Italian physician, who discovered them. Their function is to convey the human egg from the ovaries (the organs where it is developed) to the womb. To convey a distinct idea of the formation of these tubes and their relations to the womb, let us imagine the trunk of a man parted from head and neck, and separated from the pelvis at the waist; the fallopian tubes would be represented by the two arms spread right and left, even to the ends of the fingers. Let us imagine the cavity of the trunk to be continued through the arms, to the center of the palm of the hand, and we have a figure, which, although much larger in proportion, is not unlike that of the womb with its fallopian tubes. Now, to complete the similitude, let us imagine a string, starting from the armpit and hanging loosely by one of the fingers of the outstretched hand. On this string, somewhat nearer the hand than the armpit let there be a little bag containing from ten to twenty grains, from the size of a pin's head to a pea; this bag represents an ovary; and we thus have a complete representation of the womb and its appendages.

Each fallopian tube is about four inches in length, having a canal, exceedingly minute, but which gradually widens into a trumpet-shaped extremity. Its outer end terminates in fringe-like processes (the fingers of the above figure), to one of which is connected the outer end of the ovary. Here we are reminded again of the hand in a semiflex condition, making of the palm a hollow whenever so required for the reception of an egg that has parted from the ovary.

It is physiologically stated, that once a month one of these eggs bursts from its prison in the ovary, and makes its way to the fimbriated or fringed end of the fallopian tube, where it is received and held, and, through a vibratory motion of these fringes, pushed forward through the whole length of the fallopian tube, to the cavity of the womb.

The ovaries are elongated, oval-shaped bodies, situated on the string already described, on each side of the womb. They are about an inch and one-half in length, three-quarters of an inch in thickness, and weigh from an eighth to a quarter of an ounce. They contain the so-called "Graafian" vesicles or cells, each enclosing an egg. As already stated, each ovary is supplied with ten or twenty of these vesicles, varying in size according to their state of development.

The ovum, or egg, is a small spherical body, situated near the center of the immature graafian vesicle, gradually approaching its walls as the vesicle matures. When ripe, the vesicle yields, leaving the egg free. Compared with the common knowledge regarding eggs of fowls or fishes, one might suppose that the human egg would in size be proportionate to those of the above-mentioned animals. But this is far from being the case, as the human egg is so minute that it would take two or three hundred in a line to make an inch in length. In fact they are so small that they are not detected by the naked eye, and the assistance of a microscope is required to discover and examine them.

CHAPTER VIII.

THE BREASTS.

THE Breasts are classified by anatomists and physiologists among the generative organs of woman; and properly so, for their development and functions are simultaneous with those of the organs already described. The sympathy and relation between them are so intimate, that one is hardly affected without the other. While the womb retains and nourishes the offspring for nine months, the breasts are preparing to fulfill the same duty of supplying nutrition to the child for a year or more after it shall have left its internal abode in its mother's womb, to enter upon that outer life where it is to grow according to its species for the completion of the mission assigned to it.

The breasts are two in number; hemispherical in shape, representing a flattened cone with the base upon the chest. They are rudimentary in man, and in the young girl, but become developed in the latter at the period of her puberty. Their size and shape vary in different individuals and in women of different races. They also vary in weight and dimensions at different periods of life and under different circumstances. They increase during pregnancy, and especially after delivery, and become wasted away in old age. The left breast is generally a little larger than the right.

On the outer surface, and just below the center, is a

small conical prominence named "the nipple," which is of darker color than the surface of the breast, and is surrounded by a circle called "areola" having also a deeper tint than the surrounding skin. The shades of color of both the areola and the nipple vary according to the complexion of the subject, being of a delicate rosy hue in blondes, and much darker in brunettes. This color is of importance, inasmuch as it is affected by pregnancy, providing a reliable sign by which the physician determines whether the woman is in a state of pregnancy or not.

The dimensions and shape of the nipples vary also in different individuals, in some women being very slightly developed, in others very largely, while in some they are so small as to hardly come to the surface of the breast. The nipple is traversed from base to summit by lactiferous ducts, fifteen or twenty in number, which open by as many minute orifices near the free extremity of the organ. The breasts contain each a "mammary gland," properly so called. This gland is divided into several lobes and has the appearance of a bunch of grapes. Each lobe is composed of an aggregation of a number of lobules, like grapes attached to small stems. This ramification of small stems unite in five or six principal ones which end at the nipple. The lobules secrete the milk, and the stems are the lactiferous ducts that convey it to the nipple.

A proportionately well developed breast is an ornament to woman's figure. A well defined throat, blending with the elliptical lines of a well rounded breast, add grace and attraction to her chest. It is not only a beauty of presence, but one suggestive of perfection in the attributes of woman in her relation to maternity. Woman without a breast is seldom prolific, and furnishes no food to her offspring. The want of development of these organs is more often due to mismanagement than to constitutional causes. Poor, laboring women are seldom deficient in them; fashionable women are seldom in possession of well developed ones. Why? Girls, who from an early period assist their parents in the daily labor of self-sustenance, exercise their arms, the muscles of the chest generally—while ladies' daughters are engaged in trifling occupations which require but a moderate motion of their fingers. It requires more than finger-work to favor an expansion of the chest, and an elevation of all the muscles that cover it. The "Pectoralis Major," which, more than other muscle, is engaged in every motion of the chest, is inserted in the upper part of the arm; every flex or reflex action of the arm, in pulling, or lifting, is accomplished with the assistance of that muscle. As muscular exercise is conducive to muscular development, it follows that the girl who kneads her bread, sweeps her floor, makes her bed, digs in her garden, lifts books, chairs and tables, or otherwise works in her household, has a better chance for a full, well-rounded chest and throat, than the girl whose vocation is at the writing desk, or who spends her precious time at playing with the tips of her fingers in her attempts to force an unwilling needle through silk or cashmere.

The above paragraph is not intended as an appeal to vanity, but to a just conception of strength, health and beauty. A chest well covered with muscles, and even with fat, is better protected from climatic vicissitudes, from cold and dampness, than the poor, thin, undeveloped one, that every breath of air threatens with coughs and pulmonary irritations.

If the mandates of fashionable society are such as to dishonor the home-labor that has been the pride of our grandmothers, it is evident that something must be done in place of it, to secure the health of the children of these elegant devotees of fashion and mannerism.

Sad as it may seem, there are mothers who see more dignity in the swinging of dumb-bells than in kneading bread; others that consider pulling oneself up by rings or ropes a fitter employment for a lady-like girl than the lifting of a mattrass, or tucking in bed-covers; others, in fact, who think it more refined to play than to work.

It might be in vain to tell these ladies that their girls would lose nothing, but gain a great deal, morally, if, in the exercise for their health, they would accomplish something in the way of necessary labor that otherwise must be done and paid for.

Not professing to give a moral lecture on this subject, but to encourage all women in securing health and strength for their daughters, we will agree that if they will not work, they must play. For such, then, as find no comfort or attraction in home duties, we would suggest that their pleasures be of a nature that will otherwise supply to them the amount of exercise necessary to healthful growth and luxuriant development. For this purpose we would suggest rowing, tossing balls, croquet, quoits, graces, at seasons when such exercises can be performed without exposure to inclemency of weather, or to high and low temperatures. At other times, girls might attend well-regulated schools of gymnastics. In connection with these exercises, it should not be forgotten that open air contributes that important element, oxygen, which stimulates the circulation, increases vitality, and supplies the decarbonizing agent of the body.

The mammary glands within the breasts, like all the generative organs, remain dormant until the evolution of puberty, when they at once respond to the general excitation of the system. Their lobes become more and more voluminous, and the arterial circulation within them more active. Consequently the breasts then enlarge in proportion, and become very sensitive, in sympathy with the uterine organs, which now, for the first time, give evidence of life. From this time forward the breasts will be subject to monthly changes. They will swell and harden, become tender to the touch, and be the seat at times of prickly sensations and fugitive pains. Even the nipples and the areola surrounding them will assume a deeper shade of color, and be subject to erections.

The development of these organs will now be gradual, but continuous, until the age of eighteen, when woman seems to have attained a stage of completeness in all her organs. It is during this period of growth that care should be taken not to interfere with its progress, and when everything calculated to bear with undue pressure upon those organs should be avoided. It is well known that pressure on soft tissue will induce absorption and absolute diminution of volume. Pressure in this case will also prevent the deposit of adipose tissue, which is thrown around the glands for their protection, and which gives the breast roundness, grace of form, and delicacy of texture; it also prevents the growth of the glands whose functions are so important in the mother. Pressure will rob the breasts of that elevation which imparts beauty to the contour of woman's bust, and flatten them into a shapeless mass. It will compress the nipples, thus rendering nursing difficult, painful, and even perhaps impossible.

A finely developed breast needs no mechanical support; but a gentle support, without pressure, may be allowed in cases of excessive development.

The grace and symmetry of a good figure is not determined by a contracted waist, but by well developed chest and breasts. A flat, narrow chest is not handsome, and all the cunning of the art of skilled dress-makers cannot improve it. On the contrary, the devices used by these fashionable moulders tend only to diminish the already diminutive organs. Padding is only a form of compression, and cannot fail to induce absorption and prevent expansion.

We have dwelt on this subject to impress upon girls the physiological necessities which are required both to preserve their health and to add to their beauty, which is an element of success in their field of struggle.

The young girl, who, as has been said, "Heretofore was but an equivocal being, without sex," henceforth becomes *woman*, recognized as such, by the symmetrical development of her body, by the perfection of her proportions and elegance of form, by the delicacy of her features, by the harmony of her voice, by her sensibilities and affections; nay, by her character, tastes, disposition, and habits, and even by her maladies.

A metamorphosis has taken place, striking, but attractive, that puts her at the head of creation in all that is beautiful and lovely. She enters upon her life-work already a conqueror, winning all around her by the glance of her eye, by the tenderness of her heart, by the fertility of her brain, and by the noble inspiration of her soul.

CHAPTER IX.

TEMPERAMENTS.

THE GUIDE FOR MORAL AND PHYSICAL EDUCATION.

A KNOWLEDGE of individual temperament is indispensable to a correct understanding of individual cases, and to the formation of proper judgment in administering to their wants. A mechanic must know his metal before he can select the instruments for his work. To the housewife a cloth is a cloth, truly; but before treating it to a wash, she will be sure to observe whether it be of silk, of linen, or of cotton. Experience has taught her that the same treatment will not suit them all; that under it, one would shrink, while another would stretch; one retain its color, another fade. In other words, her practical good sense would suggest such treatment as is suited to the peculiar material of the cloth.

Without fear of offending the dignity of the medical profession, we will liken the physician to that sensible person. "One man's meat is another man's poison," is an old proverb. Experience has taught the fact; science has endeavored to explain it. A person is a person, indeed; but wherein one person differs from another requires the closest and most earnest investigation before one can suggest and administer remedial agencies intended to preserve the integrity of the health, or procure its recovery when once lost.

It is on account of this truth, and not of professional vanity or personal interests, that physicians universally condemn the nostrums advertised by conceited donkeys and venal conjurors to cure specific diseases. To the thinker, this baneful practice is a mystery of our civilization. Rivers of treacherous mixtures, and tons of illy adapted pills, emblazoned with the subtle devices and impudent pretensions of covetousness, find their way into the delicate human stomach, which, if it had voice, would give a shriek of horror that would reach the innermost recesses of the inhabited earth. The only apology that can be made for this foolhardiness is, that when man is sick, he is also so mentally deteriorated as to be unable to resist the baited offer, which, in a healthy condition, he would perceive to contain nothing but the cupidity of the inventor. No person is qualified to suggest a treatment for disease who is not thoroughly acquainted with all its symptoms, and with all predisposing causes derived from the temperament of the patient as well.

Temperament is defined by Dunglison as follows: "The peculiar mental and physical character of an individual, arising from the relations and proportions between the constituent parts of the body; natural organization or constitution." Hufeland says: "Constitutions or temperaments establish among men profound distinctions, by which not only the sense of the inner life, but also its relation with the exterior, through which it is influenced, are affected in a different manner. And whether it is in the humors, in the solids, or in the mind, as medical men from the earliest periods have contended, it avails but little; for forces of matter are so intimately connected that one determines the other, and that in certain organizations man will be predisposed to certain maladies, his reason and mental disposition to a particular tendency, and when such an organization is congenital [born with the person] its manifestations will last for the whole life."

The question of temperaments engaged the attention of philosophers in the earliest times of the Romans and the Greeks. The many discussions and treatises on the subject by learned men, although showing various and even contradictory opinions as to causes, nevertheless confirm the reality of its existence, and the importance of understanding it.

Temperaments have been classified and sub-classified, until they reach the number of fifteen or more, but it will suffice the purpose of this book to treat of the following classification: the *sanguine*, the *lymphatic*, the *bilious*, the *nervous*, and the *mixed.*

SANGUINE TEMPERAMENT.

The external manifestation of the sanguine temperament is described by Hufeland as follows, "Its prominent character is, great and changeable excitability, impressionable by all that causes mental or physical irritation. A person possessed of this temperament is fond of gaiety and the pleasures of life; he is predisposed to good humor, politeness and sociability; he is distinguished by good intentions, but also by lack of perseverance and firmness. Physically his blood circulates freely and is reproduced easily, even after great loss of it; his tendency is plethora and congestion. His heart and lungs are the most vulnerable organs; he is more liable to inflammatory diseases than to chronic:

the crisis in disease is easy; altogether it is a good temperament."

One endowed with this temperament should avoid all sources of irritation, stimulating drinks, excessive, fatigue, violent passions, the heat of the sun, warm and confined atmospheres. Vegetable food and water should be the greatest portion of his dietary. De Ponsan properly says: "The woman of sanguine temperament thrives better in a temperate atmosphere than in a dry and changeable one. While she should dress herself according to atmospheric vicissitudes, she will not need heavy garments, but uniformity in their application. She should bathe in water not too hot nor too cold. In her diet she should eschew succulent and copious animal food, particularly when highly seasoned; all wines, liquors, coffee and tea. In summer she should temper her thirst by slightly acidulated beverages; should take moderate exercise, attend to her excretions, occupy herself in work that does not excite the mind or inflame the imagination." Her exercise, although moderate, should be continuous; for muscular activity, if not excessive, prevents engorgement of blood. She should avoid heated rooms, and live in well ventilated apartments, to prevent determination of blood to the head. In this manner she will be free from the congestive headaches so common in plethoric women. Her menstruation will be copious and highly colored.

LYMPHATIC TEMPERAMENT.

The lymphatic temperament may be said to be the opposite of the sanguine, being characterized by want of sensibility and by inertia. The reactions either of sickness or of mental disturbance are scarcely ever violent. "The intellectual faculties are not easily impressed or excited into action; comprehension is slow, and undertakings are not entered into with avidity. Indeed, it may be said that a general state of torpidity pervades both the moral and the physical." Persons of this temperament are liable to catarrhal diseases, to obstructions of the intestines, to muscular relaxation, and obesity; their appearance is characterized by red or blonde hair of fine texture, blue eyes, white and velvety skin, soft flesh, pale lips, and often by a considerable development of nose, lips, ears, hands, and feet.

Women of this temperament are generally affected by that discharge of white mucus called leucorrhœa.

The regimen for lymphatic temperaments should be to force the general inertia into activity; hence walking, riding, boating, out-door games, and even gymnastics should be resorted to frequently. "The diet forbidden in the sanguine temperament would be very appropriate in the lymphatic." To such a temperament a shock, even a misfortune, may prove sanitary for the exertion that it may inspire. Persons thus constituted should cultivate cheerful company, occupation, or amusements, travel, or occupy themselves in anything that promotes energy, both corporal and mental.

Ponsan, a hygienic philosopher, suggests for persons, and particularly for women, of this temperament, "a dry atmosphere, well lighted and well aired habitations, warm clothing, a moderate use of cold baths, stimulating food, such as well-seasoned meats, a moderate use of good wine, little coffee, and all diaphoretic beverages having the power to increase perspiration. The skin to be kept active by dry friction and the muscular system by exercise, and not too much sleep."

Such persons, having regard for the regimen above described, should be careful in not being too liberal in taking medicaments calculated to debilitate by loss of blood, by purging or otherwise. A visit to the country abounding in ozone, exercise on horseback, boating, outdoor games, hunting, &c., will greatly assist in the promotion of that vigor so necessary to the already torpid constitution.

BILIOUS TEMPERAMENT.

The liver and the biliary apparatus seem to be peculiarly sensitive, and easily excited to endure activity in this temperament.

"Persons thus organized are generally passionate, violent, given to anger. Impulsive, they will undertake things with more ardor than prudence, act with great precipitation, and, therefore, are capable of heroism or of evil. Physically they are of brown complexion, their hair is black, the skin hard, and the muscles dry. Pathologically they are predisposed to an abundant secretion of bile, and to all diseases depending upon biliary derangements; to sanguinous congestions, to inflammations; such diseases appearing almost always in a violent manner. Persons of such organization should be educated to conquer their irascibility and their passionate disposition, by a proper and timely appeal to their reason, which is not defective in intellectual strength. They should be taught to cultivate the affections, for it is through them that they may possibly be able to curb the vehemence of their temper." They should avoid contentions and litigations, and all occurrences likely to lead to warm discussions. Their diet should be drawn from the vegetable rather than from the animal kingdom; they should not indulge in stimulating beverages, but make free use of acids—either in water or otherwise. They should eat plenty of fruit, attend carefully to their excretions, and never allow themselves to become constipated.

It is in this temperament that physical exercise is particularly demanded. A sedentary life is baneful; while open air activity is pre-eminently healthful. Systematic cold bathing and dry frictions will also contribute to their comfort.

NERVOUS TEMPERAMENT.

This temperament is common among women. It is detected in persons of "lean and dry complexions, small development of muscle, an expressive and changeable countenance, a brilliant eye, high forehead, quick movement They receive impressions quickly and strongly, exhibit an energy often disproportionate to their strength, often depressed without commensurate reason. The distinctive signs of this temperament are: quickness of motion, mobility of expression, intellectual vigor, excessive activity of the sympathies, and proneness to the animal passions."

A woman thus organized should be habituated to systematic labor and occupation. She should breathe a temperate atmosphere, but rather moist; live in valleys rather than mountains; near the water rather than in elevated localities. Her bath should be tepid; her diet of young meats and gelatine, of fruits, and everything digestible, precluding spices, alcohol, and, particularly, tea and coffee. A little wine may not be inadmissible, but her beverage should be water, sometimes tempered with mucilaginous substances. Exercise should never be carried to excess, for the reaction would be weakness. She should refrain from the stimulation of her passions, seeking calmness and uniformity of life. She should avoid all that is calculated to excite the nervous system, and, particularly, all that over-stimulates the intellectual faculties and immoderately excites the sympathies. '*Moderation* ought to be the motto that is to guide her in all her thoughts, feelings and actions." (Ponsan.)

The nervous system is self-consuming; hence persons in whom this constitutional trait predominates should add no preventable excitements, in order to avoid a too early consumption of vital force.

MIXED TEMPERAMENTS.

The temperaments are not always so distinct as described. There are persons in whom two of the above named temperaments are apparently mixed, and they are then denominated as sanguine-nervous, lymphatico-nervous, bilious-nervous, bilious-sanguine, etc.

When this is the case, the hygienic treatment should be selected according to the combination as found.

It has already been stated that the nervous temperament predominates among women, and as this work is especially dedicated to them, a further expression of its necessities may not be superfluous.

When the utero-generative system is endowed with excessive sensibility, "it should be calmed by regimen adapted to nervous temperament, and by the avoidance *in childhood* of all that might stimulate precocious desires. In the adult, all that disposes to amorous passions, to suspicious attachments, to questionable dramas or pictures, to free conversations, and to all spectacular representations of doubtful propriety. When, however, apathy predominates in the generative system, strengthening diets, horseback riding, boating, walking, stimulating baths should be adopted."

This sketch of temperaments, although necessarily superficial, should be carefully considered by everyone having the charge of children; for if the modification of natural propensities is possible, through systematic hygiene, it is possible only during the elastic period of youth. Age hardens these predispositions into permanency. The experienced husbandman trains his young trees before they attain such proportions and such strength as to have become unwieldy; so the educator should early and carefully examine the predominant inclinations of pupils, lest they become inured to ways that are crooked, and habits that are disastrous. Proper management in time often saves young people from indulgences that are inconsistent with health and happiness.

It is especially for girls that we plead, as their nervous susceptibility is greater. City life and the habits of people of affluence are those of indulgence, not only in the epicurism of the table, but also in surcharging the imagination. It is no wonder, then, that physicians find much occupation among this class of women, who are generally affected by diseases sprung from a too early demand upon their vitality. "Female diseases," vulgarly so called, are more common among these than among women inhabiting the country. Puberty comes to them sooner; so does child-bearing; so do uterine affections; so does old age; so does death. Confined to heated rooms, devoted to tyrannical fashion, stimulated by too early and complex studies; drinking tea, coffee, and wines; eating meats, spices, and gravies; reading romantic literature; attending the theater and the ball room; exposed to vanity and allurements of every kind, the girl, like a plant, is forced into an early flowering season and premature decay. Many of the practicing physicians would be compelled to find employment in other pursuits, were it not for the headaches, backaches, debility; the congestions, ulcerations and displacements of the womb; the irregular or painful menstruation; the lung troubles, that abound among the women of populous cities.

The proof that these natural temperaments are modified by education and habits is found in the fact that certain temperaments prevail in certain countries, while they do not prevail in others. Locality, social condition, and climate have as much relation to those modifications as habits, diet, &c. Thus, in the United States, the nervous temperament predominates; while in Germany the lymphatic, in Italy the sanguine, prevail.

Wealth is also, in part, responsible for these physiological deviations. The abuse of stimulants in this abounding land is greatly due to the ability of every man to purchase them. Dyspepsia, so common in America, and which drives so many of our citizens to Europe in quest of health, is greatly due to the large and rich provisions of the American table. Thousands of American women, permanent valetudinarians, would enjoy uninterrupted health if the luxuries and comforts of life were not so easily obtained; if occupation were a necessity, and the use of coffee, tea and stimulating diets were impossible. Women that can ride do not walk; those that are allowed to kill time by reading romances do not work. The sun, that revivifying element of our creation, is shunned, because it bronzes their pallid complexion, the wind because it chaps their skin, labor because it enlarges their hands; and all this, because they have money to pay menials to do their work and obey their behests. Wealth will deteriorate the physical nature of the American people as it has done that of other nations before them.

In nations where large populations exist and wealth is greatly subdivided, these luxuries are impossible, and their people enjoy the benefit of the deprivation. Their habitations are kept cool through inability to provide fuel; and the same reason renders them prudent in the provision of the table, and less indulgent in those social pleasures which, when carried to excess, lead to disturbances in the human economy. Under that stringency, however forced upon them by circumstances, they grow healthy and strong, and are seldom affected by chronic ailments.

CHAPTER X.

PUBERTY:

THE THRESHOLD OF WOMANHOOD.

THE course of human life has by physiologists and psychologists been divided into four stages, namely: Infancy, Adolescence, Virility, Dementia.

This division is somewhat arbitrary, for the exact lines of demarcation are imaginary at best. That there are in life periods sufficiently distinct to be appreciated by the intellect of man, there is no doubt; but exactly where they commence and end, it is as impossible to tell as to fix the dividing line between two States without a positive knowledge of the topography, and of the measurements of limitation. Yet a traveller, in a train of cars running from New York to San Francisco, although not able to tell exactly where and when he crosses the boundary line between State and State, will observe from time to time a difference in the architectural style of dwellings, in the dress, manner and pursuits of the people, sufficient to suggest to his mind that, in the progress of his travels, he has crossed boundaries between States, or sections of the country. He has met no sentry and no custom house officer at each border to startle him into a knowledge of such fact, because, although the States are many, the country is one; yet his intelligence and power of observation have gradually brought him into that consciousness of change, which upon inquiry he is assured to be really a transition from one State to another. So it is in the long run of life; there is no distinct line of demarcation between one stage and another; but, unconsciously to us, these changes pass under our eyes, until an occurrence, even of trifling importance, makes us aware that the girl of fifteen thinks and acts differently from what she did, or would have done, at ten. We moreover become aware, as our mind is awakened to this fact, that this change is not transient, but, on the contrary, positive and permanent. Her demands, her necessities, have undergone real modifications, and the physiologist and psychologist mark this as a new era, just as the traveller decides in his own mind that he has truly entered a new dominion.

These periods or stages of life are observed not only in man, but in all living things, vegetable as well as animal. A seed is planted, exposed to moisture and heat that excite its latent life into activity, and soon a plant rises from the earth; for a certain length of time this will grow; for another it will bloom, and for another it will yield fruit; then bear seed after its own kind, decay and perish. All the changes between birth and death occur, in some plants, in a short season of three months. It is the same with some animalculæ and worms. The silk worm, for instance, will, in the short space of six weeks start from its condition of egg-existence and go through all the vicissitudes of life, propagation and death. In this short time it was brought forth, matured, spun a large quantity of silk, passed a season of torpitude in chrysalis, was metamorphosed into a moth, entered into its connubial state, reproduced thousands after its own kind, and died. But amidst this ephemeral life, we find the oak of the forest, the pine of the mountains, and the cedar, undergoing all these changes (except those of birth and death), and being renewed annually in vigor, during a long life of centuries.

The changes that occur, classifiable into periods, are not all alike in manner, or in length of time, either in the animal or vegetable kingdoms. In man they are less sudden or salient than in plants, or other animals; neither is there a broken link in the progression to suggest the moment for mark. At times, however, the mind is arrested by an expression, or by a word, significant and startling, that leads one to realize the fact that under his very eye a creature has passed from one state to another, or has freed itself from the thraldom of childhood and advanced to a higher degree of dignity. If through stupidity you fail to recognize this fact, you are quickly made aware of it from the demeanor of the person concerned. Although your dullness may not provoke resentment in the young person so carelessly unobserved, it may, nevertheless, incite an expression of self-appreciation, which you cannot fail to notice and respect. Henceforward you accept the fact that a change has occurred, and that you are addressing a person who has entered into a higher state of mental and physical development.

We have mentioned four periods of life, which, on reflection, bear resemblance to the four seasons of the year. Philosophically, as well as poetically, it would not be inappropriate to call Infancy, *spring;* Adolescence, *summer;* Virility, *autumn;* Dementia, *winter.*

From our work on *Maternity* we will transfer to these

pages a brief and concise delineation of these seasons of human life.

"*Infancy*, or childhood, is a period almost totally vegetative; it is a period of growth of the organs before the mind is sufficiently developed to influence and control them, ere they are ready for action. This period will embrace twelve or fourteen years of our life.

"*Adolesence* is the progression of the former period. The term comes from the Latin *adolescere* (to grow, to become strong). It denotes that period of human life between the first signs of puberty and the time when the body ceases to grow, and has acquired all its physical perfection. This period commences at eleven or twelve years of age with women, and at fourteen and fifteen with men; ending with the former at twenty-one, with the latter at twenty-five years of age, or thereabout.

"The changes that the organism undergoes at this epoch of life are very remarkable in both sexes. . . .

"In the *woman*, those physical and moral changes are not less remarkable [than in man]. The organ of her especial function, the womb, which so far has given no sign of existence, comes out of its state of inertia; the menses appear, to return periodically every month; the breasts, whose functional existence is so intimately connected with the womb, commence to develop; every organ perfects itself, in preparation for the process of reproduction. The body of the woman, however, retains some of that infantile delicacy of texture, of that suppleness, of that grace of movement, which constitute the great contrast with the striking vigor, the activity, the impetuosity that distinguishes the same stage in man.

"*Virility*, 'manhood,' is the period that follows *ado-*

lescence, and ends with old age. In the age of manhood, the body has acquired all its proportions. The life becomes more even and uniform; the ideas, which have followed in the ratio of physical development, now become more profound and fixed, and the movements of the body consonant with the dignity of the mind. The time of brilliant illusions has passed; imagination gives place to judgment, frivolity to circumspection, heat of passion to reason, vivacity to reflection, impulsive generosity to prudence and calculation, and aimless recklessness to sagacity and ambition.

"*Dementia* is the period when the body and the mind decay. It is less distinct, as it varies in different people according to the preservation of their health; and oftentimes we see an active mind in a decayed body. Yet it is a period that must come sooner or later to both mind and body."

Of all these periods we have to treat only of that which relates to *Adolescence in Woman;* for it is with the intention of guarding and preserving her during this important part of her life that this work has been undertaken, because then it is that her moral habits are forming, and her organs are shaping themselves to a fashion, *in which they must remain ever after*. It is during this time, also, that the mind, heretofore passive and almost totally imitative, springs as from itself into an existence of self-dependence, self-regulation, and gives evidence of originality of thought and conception. All the senses become more active; and one can notice the human being gradually breaking away from the anchor of parental control, and drifting towards the current of life, where it will thenceforth steer its own course.

It is also in the time of adolescence that latent diseases often develop themselves; and the offspring of parents who have died of tuberculous consumption need now the greatest attention, for in this condition of susceptibility, the slightest indiscretion is often the spark that kindles a fatal fire.

It is now, also, the time when one of the most important functions of woman's life becomes established; and it is imperative that its beginning, as well as its continuance, be in accord with the laws of her nature.

MENSTRUATION.

The function which characterizes the development of puberty in woman, is *"Menstruation."* Knowing, as we do, the multitude of ills, the discomforts, the weakness, the disability that may follow an imperfection of this process, we can but feel irresistibly impelled to warn the mothers, as well as the daughters, that a study of its normal type and the causes of its abnormalities, are things which should come within their perfect knowledge.

In former chapters, and in the paragraph on adolescence, we have already mentioned the moral and the external physical development of puberty. It now remains, to explain the physiological process of menstruation, to which all other functions seem subordinate, and which will occur periodically every month, from the age of about fourteen to forty-five. We may be allowed to repeat, that this phenomenon is the real sign of puberty in woman, as well as a normal indication of her development; without it her beauty would perish, and her future be involved in suffering. A regular occurrence of this function is probably the most reliable symptom of health in woman. At the age above mentioned, if nature is not obstructed in the accomplishment of its laws by any extraordinary obstacle, woman will not fail to become subject to this menstrual revolution.

Warning symptoms. The menstrual eruption may be anticipated by a sense of weight below the small of the back, extending away down into the pelvic basin; by an unusual sensation of heat in the genitals; by fugitive pains; by general lassitude; by an excitability of the nervous system depriving the individual even of sleep; by heat; by slight pains and heavy feelings in the head; by oppressed respiration, and highly colored urine.

The breasts increase in volume and sensibility, becoming even painful to the touch. The pulse quickens, and the circulation becomes so active as to give a new expression to the face, and brilliancy to the eyes. The digestive functions often become deranged, and the appetite depraved or made unnatural.

It is not uncommon, while these functions are preparing in the young girl, to find that she is tormented by strange tastes, such as a desire to eat clay, slate-pencils, charcoal, salt, pickles, etc. She may soon be affected by incontinence of urine; diarrhœa or constipation; sweats, often offensive; feverishness; spasmodic and nervous affections such as neuralgia; quivering or contractions of muscles, etc.

A girl of nervous-sanguine temperament, of an imaginative turn of mind, may be disturbed in her sleep by frightful dreams that awaken her suddenly. Even her moral disposition seems quickly to change, being now easily affected by impressions, irritated by the slightest opposition to her wishes—or she may be overwhelmed by sadness, breaking out in tears and sobs, followed by hysterical laughs, and even convulsions. She seems not able to control her passions of love or anger; she changes from one state of mind to another, with quickness and without cause, and actually becomes an object of anxiety to her parents and her friends. This unnatural state may occur, from time to time, for a month or two, or sometimes longer, before the first appearance of the menstrual flow; and it is observed that as soon as the flow commences, and in proportion to its continuance, these symptoms of vital irritation diminish, and finally cease with the flow at the end of the third or fourth day.

There are instances, however, where the premonitory symptoms are still more severe. The process in these severe cases is often preceded by a serous or watery discharge from the womb; by spasmodic cough; by cutaneous eruptions, such as those red, tingling and itching spots, commonly called *hives;* by violent colics, by great nervous depression, and by a greenish (chlorotic) hue in the complexion.

The presence of these symptoms would naturally lead one to suppose that a serious malady exists, requiring the interference of the medical man; and we would not say that his assistance may not often be necessary to calm the apprehensions of the patient, and the attendants, and to suggest some mild means to give relief from actual suffering; but we nevertheless desire to make clear the fact that patience, quietude, and the free flow of menstrual fluid, will dissipate all the previous irritations, and bring the patient back to her normal state.

The establishment of this function oftentimes produces a most salutary effect on girls that have heretofore suffered with chronic affections, relieving them, as if by magic, of troubles which had been believed to be permanent.

These morbid conditions are not necessary concomitants of the preparatory stage in the evolution of this function; for it does happen that girls are overtaken by the coming of menstruation, without being conscious of having undergone any of the above described morbid states; although flashes of heat, flushes in the face, heaviness of the head, and slight nervous excitability, may have occurred without creating any marked impression.

The first appearance of the menses generally occurs as follows: On the first day there will be a flow of a fluid, something like blood and water mixed, which will occur at intervals. On the second day, the fluid is less watery, and the flow more continuous. On the third day it will be almost pure blood, that will flow without interruption. On the fourth day the flow diminishes quite perceptibly, and is interrupted at times. On the fifth day it again assumes quite a watery appearance, coming at intervals, greatly diminished in quantity; until it entirely ceases. Now all the previous symptoms disappear, and the girl, well and buoyant, may be satisfied that she has actually entered the most interesting period of her life.

CHAPTER XI.

MENSTRUATION;

ITS PHILOSOPHY AND PHYSIOLOGY.

ON superficial inquiry one might suppose menstruation to be nothing more than a troublesome and unnecessary process. But, scientifically speaking, it would be a heresy to declare this, or any other process of nature, unnecessary; for scientists have long since learned that all the requirements of nature are absolutely unavoidable for the accomplishment of the intent of the Creator. This truth should rather be a cause of pleasure to man, who would then know that his own organization, as well as all surrounding him, is not the result of accident or of fortuitous circumstances, but a part of a grand whole in the creation.

Nothing is left to chance in nature; and this troublesome function in the life of woman is not unnecessary, but a useful and important law of her being. Our duty is to study and understand the import of that law, that she may be able to abide by its restrictions, and become an active agent in its preservation.

What, then, is Menstruation? To explain it, philosophers and scientists have invaded the innermost sources of its origin, and through observation, experiment, comparison, have arrived at logical inferences that are accepted to-day as a satisfactory explanation of its existence.

Its *periodicity* first attracted their attention, and then they found that other animals and living things were subject to similar periodicity for purposes of reproduction. Reproduction, then, became foremost in their inquiries; and the more they studied and reflected upon the subject the more they became convinced that the process of menstruation had relation to it. Then came various theories, more or less plausible, in proportion to to the advancement in the science of anatomy and physiology.

It is not many years since science was in great obscurity; indeed, it is only within this last century that great strides have been made in the knowledge of functional and anatomical organization. It is not, therefore, surprising, that great ignorance still exists in this regard, and that obsolete theories yet continue to prevail in the minds of the uneducated and the vulgar.

We will pass over the period when the products of the menstrual flux were believed to be a curse that would wither and blemish everything they touched. The advancement of science, literature and art of centuries has, from constant research into causes and effects, emancipated the human mind from many a superstition, among which this was one of the most flagrant.

Physiologists tell us now that menstruation is a part of the process for the propagation of our own species. It might properly be called ovulation, or the development and discharge of the egg, or germ of human life. It is found that when the ovaries are absent, through accident or congenital malformation, menstruation does not occur. It has also been found in cases of the death of a nubile woman, and of other animals, while menstruation is in progress, that the ovaries were in process of giving birth to an ovum (an egg).

Before proceeding further in the perusal of this chapter, the reader should become acquainted with the articles on the womb and ovaries already given; for without knowledge of the construction and relation of those organs, their functions may not be easily understood.

Sentimental people affect to believe themselves spiritual beings, and seem to be overcome by a sense of degradation whenever reminded that they are associated with an animal nature. These specimens of human vanity feel lowered at the very thought of the affiliation of their moral nature with the crude, ponderous, and brute matter of the purely animal. But unfortunately for those who are thus afflicted, these romantic conceptions are not in accordance with the laws that govern them. Their nature is a mixed one—the animal and the spiritual so intimately connected, that one exists by reason of the other.

Separate the spirit from the body, the union of both constituting one being, and quickly the latter resolves itself into elementary gases, through the physical laws that regulate all matter.

In the exposition of our subject, and particularly in the one that immediately follows, we are to treat of functions that are common to all animals, however inferior, viewed in the light of our elevated notion of humanity. This should not deter even the sentimentalist from giving them her closest attention.

Ovulation is not a process peculiar to the human female. It is rather an universal system of propagation in all animals. A germ is a necessity to a new being in the animal, as well as in the vegetable kingdom. In the vegetable, it is enclosed in the seed; in the animal, in the egg. There exists the closest analogy between these two systems of propagation. These facts having been established, the modes as to time and manner have been inquired into, and the result of the investigations has been to demonstrate that in the vegetable kingdom the fructified seed leaves its maternal plant, to fall to the earth, where at the proper season, and under favorable conditions, such as moisture and heat, it germinates, buds, spreads its roots, and follows in the ways of its progenitors. In the animal kingdom, some of its species deposit their eggs in places safe and favorable to their hatching. The parents of some of these sit on them, to infuse warmth into them during the time required for sufficient development to enable them to force themselves out of their shells. Others retain the egg, to hatch within an apparatus (the womb) peculiar to their kind, and thus nourish the new being within their own body, until it is so far formed and developed as to be born without danger to its life.

Plants have seeding seasons of longer or shorter duration; some having more than one season a year, others only one in a hundred years; some propagating millions after their own kind in one season, others but one. Some give maturity to their seed in one day, others in months. So with the animal kingdom. Animals have seasons of ovulation of longer or shorter duration, some bearing every day, like the hen; some once in three years, like the elephant. Some bear millions at a time, like the herring; others five or six at one brood. Some invariably two, like the pigeon; others only one, like the horse. All developing after their own kind, some are born in a few days; others in as many weeks; others in months; others in years—the new-born following always the physical laws that govern the parent in its lineage.

Hence the naturalist has divided these kingdoms into classes, classes into species, etc., for it was found that nature was intent on their continuation by constant and uniform reproduction.

Mankind is not an exception to this system; and, like other races, forms a single species, subordinate to its own laws.

At the age of puberty—namely, when the human being has acquired sufficient strength and development for procreation—the human female is subject to an evolution of eggs. The ovaries are the organs provided for the formation of these eggs. They mature monthly, one at a time, at which period the egg leaves its place of birth for its first journey on the road to life; bursts its shell (called the graafian vesicle), and is free. Helpless, however, it lies till the fringed end of the fallopian tubes goes to its assistance, grasps it in its protective cavity, and by its peculiar motion pushes the egg forward into the womb, its first station, where it is to remain for the period of nine months to acquire growth, shape, strength, after its own kind.

After the period of nine months' sojourn in this hospitable home, it is so far grown that from the size of a minute and formless seed it now weighs ten pounds, with all the beauty of human organization.

It is not, however, the fate of all human eggs to

develop into human beings, else in the pilgrimage of maternity every woman would probably produce thirty children. The egg of the mother alone is not sufficient for the reproduction of a human being, any more than the seed of a plant will develop into a new plant without having been made fruitful by the fertilizing *pollen* from the anthers. The egg is her share of the contribution towards this mysterious law of nature; man, her chosen companion, has also to pay his tribute to the new creation; and then, like the vegetable germ, the fructified seed is ready to develop.

[This particular subject, however, has been treated by the author in his work on *Maternity*, and he does not think its elaboration appropriate or necessary in this volume. *Maternity*, although published first, is properly a continuation of this book.]

This monthly evolution of an ovum is what is called by physiologists *ovulation*.

New formation in animals requires blood, just as much as new formation in plants requires sap. At certain seasons, therefore, once a month, a determination of blood to the ovaries occurs, to supply the needed elements for the formation of an egg. This flow of blood is directed not only to the ovaries, but to the womb as well, to prepare that organ for the reception of the new guest that may or may not develop into a new being. Should that egg, however, be unfructified, its residence in the womb will be but transient, and it will pass off unconsciously to its parent.

In this case the provision of blood, accumulated for the emergency, is of no further use, and is allowed to exude through the walls of the womb and pass away.

This flow of blood is called menstruation. Now, then, it may be understood why menstruation and ovulation are held as synonyms. That one process is consequent upon the other is so far true that where ovulation is impossible, as in the case of absence of the ovaries, menstruation never occurs.

Any extraordinary determination of blood to any part of the body causes a congestion, which if not relieved may go on to inflammation, with all its relative pains and dangers. The monthly congestion of the ovaries and womb is relieved by menstruation. Hence it is not surprising that the physician at that period insists upon such conduct on the part of the woman as will not interfere with or check this necessary exudation. Suppressed menstruation is always a cause of disease and danger. Indeed, any anomaly in this function never fails to reflect upon the system and induce great suffering. The causes that derange it are many, and often not within the young woman's knowledge; but it does also happen, to her shame and discredit, that with perfect knowledge of these causes, she, for the vain gratification of an hour, will imperil her whole life.

MENSTRUAL CRISIS.

Epoch of its Commencement and Mode of its Course.

As we have said, the first appearance of the menses is the signal of the epoch called *puberty* in woman. It is the occurrence that defines her sex by its peculiar function.

The age at which this phenomenon occurs for the first time varies according to individual temperament, climate, and mode of living. Like the germination of plants, it occurs sooner in warm than in cold regions. Heat hastens life in the animal as well as the vegetable kingdom; thus children of southern latitudes are comparatively more precocious than those of northern ones. To compensate for this disparity, however, nature, always intent upon maintaining an even balance, requires him who starts first to reach the end of his course soonest. Quicker to grow, quicker to die, seems an irresistible law. The precocity of the southerner, therefore, in the chances of life is no advantage over the northerner. Longevity should be reckoned in man, not so much by the length of his purely physical existence, as the continuance of the moral in harmony with the physical elements of his being.

In southern countries girls ordinarily reach the age of puberty from the tenth to the twelfth year; while those inhabiting temperate regions will not attain the same epoch until the twelfth or fourteenth year; and those of northern latitudes not until the fourteenth or sixteenth year, and even later. This average, however, is not absolute; for the human economy is also impressed by the circumstances that immediately surround it.

Thus the young lass of agricultural districts and of the mountains, living retired from the excitements of city life, on a simple and non-stimulating diet; mentally and physically occupied in out-door labor; her imagination unexposed to the stimulus of all kinds of literature, or of the spectacular dramas of city life, or the alluring scenes of the drawing-room and the dance, remains longer in that state of self-unconsciousness so lovely and so healthful during the stage of childhood. Her body grows in conformity with the laws of nature;

acquiring volume and strength, untrammeled by that forcing process of strong impressions upon the nervous system which hasten life to premature exhaustion. The occurrence of the menstrual crisis finds her, therefore, better prepared to perform all the requirements of her sex. Her intellectual faculties have the opportunity to thus develop in a strong and healthy body, enabling the woman to retain physical freshness and youthfulness of heart for a much longer period than her wearied and withering sister of the city. The modes of life of the country and the city girl are like the coach-road of olden times and the railroad of the modern: the motive of the one being safety, of the other speed.

The city girl, over-fed with meats, with highly seasoned viands, stimulated by coffee, tea, wines, and even sometimes liquor, is forced into an unnatural nervous activity. Exposed to early infatuations, to luxury, to indolence and confinement, to the vanity of fashion, to the admiration of self, she is quickly brought to that threshold of sensualism where are awakened thoughts that reflect upon her generative organs, which promptly respond, inducing untimely development, even beyond her physical power. To the surprise of her mother she announces her change. The mother's surprise should be one of sorrow; for this premature sensibility will weaken her constitution, even before she is prepared to assume that position in life which will constantly draw from the resources of her physical organization.

Parents and teachers should never forget that all that heats the body and inflames the imagination unduly hastens puberty in both sexes.

In this connection, education—alluding here particularly to the period of school-training—has a bearing that should not be overlooked.

The brain is the central motive-power of physical as well as moral life. The moral and the physical are reciprocal. That balance should not be disturbed, lest one preponderate over the other, for the time will surely come when both will suffer, particularly if the disturbance is incurred during that period of sensitiveness, the age of growth.

Besides, this functional period of girls is affected by their respective constitutions, their *temperaments*. These temperaments play a very important part not only in the conceptions, inspirations and actions of humanity, but also in the development of physical organizations. Where the nervous-sanguine temperament prevails, other things being equal, puberty will be manifested at the earliest epoch; in the lymphatico-sanguine it would be manifested at a later; and in the purely lymphatic at the latest of all.

Mothers should carefully reflect upon all these facts; for in the guidance of their daughters they will be of the greatest importance. It is to be regretted that too often the wise counsel of reason is smothered by a foolish yielding to fashion, and the advice of medical men and philosophers too often set aside with disdain, for the more insinuating and enticing whisperings of vanity.

The duration of the menstrual flux may extend from two to eight days; but the average, in the great majority of women, is only from four to five. It recurs every twenty-eight days, the days of sickness included; consequently, a woman in good health should menstruate thirteen times in one year, namely: *once every four weeks.*

If a woman, therefore, is taken flowing on the twenty-eighth day of one month her next menstruation should occur on the twenty-fifth of the following month, provided the previous month had thirty-one days; and on the twenty-sixth if it had only thirty days. It is a common mistake in women to think that the occurrence of the next menstruation will be due on the same day of the month as the last, while it cannot be so if its course is normal and regular. The monthly sickness occurs once every *lunar* month, not the month of the calendar. This is the general rule; but it sometimes happens that women, although in good state of health, menstruate every three weeks, and even oftener.

If menstruation has been suspended on account of sickness, or from natural causes, such as pregnancy and lactation, it will reappear at the time when it would have been due had the woman menstruated regularly without suspension. Thus, if a woman's menstruation, being due on the 30th of a certain month, had been suspended, and continued so four times after, in her calculation she should account for the three days for the months having thirty-one days, and for the two days for the months having thirty days, which in this case would probably sum up as follows: for the two long months, six days; for the two short months, four days; making a total of ten days, to be subtracted from the date at which they were first suspended; hence, in this case the next regular menstrual flux would be on the 20th of the month. This rule should be recollected, for in many instances it will serve conveniently in anticipating rightly the reappearance of the periods after months of suspension; and, perhaps importantly, as a guide where the medical man requires precise dates for his information.

This regular occurrence is, however, somewhat disturbed during the few first months of the beginning of puberty, when a girl is liable to an irregularity of months, until the natural function is established in all its normality.

In many instances, this process engenders no constitutional disturbance whatever; while in others, it is attended with heaviness and pain in the back, extending down even to the thighs; with burning urinations and heat around the genital parts. The usual expression of the face may change; the eyes be surrounded by a dark ring, and the eye-lids often puffed; the breath may be offensive, the breathing oppressed, and a general tension and hardness be felt at the lower part of the abdomen occasionally, heavy, or acute, colicky pains may supervene; nervousness will predominate, manifested by impatience, anger, weariness or sadness. Hysterical symptoms may even be superinduced, which not very rarely assume a spasmodic form. Should the above symptoms occur, particularly in a violent form, at every menstrual period, it would indicate a state of irritability, and even of inflammation, of the womb, requiring medical care.

The quantity of blood lost at each menstruation has been estimated to be about six ounces; but the flux depends so much upon individual temperament, age, regimen, moral and physical condition, upon climate and even season, that rarely two persons are found whose amount of loss is the same.

It is found to be greater in northern than in southern latitudes; less in women advanced in life, or those who have had many children, or whose abdomen is disproportionately large; less in women who lead a very active life, in those who are nourished by gross food, and in those of an impressionable imagination. It is therefore greater in women residing in cities than in those of the country. The brunette of a sanguine temperament will have a flow abundant in quantity, rich in color, and containing so much fibrine as to easily coagulate into clots. This free discharge of the sanguine temperament is often a relief to the person thus constituted. The loss will be less among those of lymphatic temperament, inclined to corpulence, to languor, and general inertia. It is particularly among those of nervous temperament that the flux is attended with pain and general discomfort; while the quantity varies, being at times copious, at others scanty, and more or less deficient in red globules.

This flux has its rise, its height, and its fall; appearing on the first day as a lightly colored discharge, increasing in red globules on the second, and reaching its height of quantity and intensity of color on the third, decreasing on the fourth, and generally disappearing on the fifth.

The periods are sometimes anticipated by a whitish mucous discharge often mistaken for leucorrhœa. They are naturally suspended during pregnancy, and for eight or nine months during lactation, or nursing. This rule is subject to but few exceptions.

During menstruation woman is very susceptible to moral impressions. All her senses are more acute, causing her to become irritable and even impetuous; unimportant occurrences, such as the unexpected and sudden appearance of a person, a message of joy or sorrow, may throw her into an uncontrollable fit of hysteria. With some girls melancholy prevails; profound sadness seems to control their usually bright and hopeful nature, and despondency, alarm, suspicion, jealousy, and even despair supplant genial and loving dispositions. As soon as the term is passed, however, the dark cloud melts away, the moral deflection disappears, and happy smiles again illuminate their faces.

Such is the history of menstruation in its *normal* course; the *abnormal* instances occurring from accidental or constitutional causes, or from disease, will be treated hereafter.

PART II.

HYGIENE FOR WOMEN.

HAVING in the former Part demonstrated the necessity for woman to be acquainted with the organization peculiar to her sex, and given an outline of the anatomy and physiology of the female organs, we shall devote this Part to the study of the fundamental principles of hygiene to be observed in the effort to preserve the normal condition of her functions. For convenience, it will be divided as follows:

    I. Hygienic generalities.
   II. Society, in its relation to the health of girls.
  III. Exercise, and its relation to bodily functions.
  IV. Food, its digestion, assimilation and absorption.
   V. Air, or the atmospherical conditions having relation to human health.
  VI. Clothing.

CHAPTER I.

HYGIENIC GENERALITIES.

THE delicate texture of woman's skin renders her more susceptible than man to the various changes of temperature, as well as of quality of atmosphere.

Extremes are always dangerous to her. Heat and cold, dryness or dampness, density or rarity, in excessive degree, are conditions of atmosphere to which she is extremely sensitive, particularly when the changes are sudden, as on our Atlantic coast. For the same reason, she is more susceptible to atmospheres containing deleterious substances, and those of a contagious and infectious character. Light, as well as pure and temperate air, is conducive to her health. Deprive her of sunlight, and she will blanch like a plant grown in the shade. Her very delicacy requires the influence of these elements, even more than stalwart man. Men will stand days in the furnace room of a steamship, naked to the waist, feeding the fiery furnace with coal, or will work their life long in the tunnels of the mines. Not so woman. Light and air are essential to her preservation.

Compare the city with the country woman; or with the one that breathes the purer and more rarified air of the mountains. Of course, every woman cannot be transferred to the mountains, but it is therefore even more the duty of man to see that she does not perish in the confinement of heated and ill-ventilated rooms.

The temperature of dwellings, modified, of course, according to climate and seasons, should never be elevated beyond sixty degrees Fahrenheit.

In North America, where wealth prevails, the commodities of life are generously supplied, and none more so than that of combustibles for heating. This indulgence is a great source of bad health to those compelled to the seclusion of home. The Southerner finds the atmosphere of a Northern dwelling well-nigh intolerable. The moderate temperature of his climate enables him to live longer in the open air, and consequently he suffers in the hot and close atmosphere of a Northern dwelling, even when the air without is below zero.

Heat, long continued, while exciting at first, must enervate at last, rendering vitality low, and the body susceptible to the variations of temperature felt from passing in and out of doors.

It is a mistaken notion that external heat is to supply the exhausted heat of the body, for were it so what would the Laplanders and Esquimaux do in the snow-houses of Iceland? Nature has provided that the oxygen of the air, in oxidizing the carbonaceous particles of the blood, shall induce heat; and that exercise, in quickening the circulation, will more rapidly send the blood to the lungs for the purpose of quickly subjecting it to that beautiful process of calorification. Hence, food, pure air, light and exercise, constitute the cardinal elements which give the necessary strength and heat to the body. In the application of these elements, reasonable moderation should always be adopted, and each element used only as a proportionate equivalent to the loss; for life has a proper standard which should not be encroached upon, either by excess or by tint.

The extraction of heat from the body in colder latitudes would very soon cause death, if carbonaceous substances, such as oils, fats, meats, etc., were not taken into the system as fuel, and converted into heat by the oxygen breathed from the air. It is the experience of all travelers in the icy regions that the diet above mentioned will preserve life when clothing or fire, the latter particularly, would fail. It is an historical fact, that the French, returning from Moscow, fared better when they kept aloof from the fire and forced themselves into motion than when they bivouacked around the campfires, resting from their fatigue. The laws of nature can hardly ever be replaced by artificial custom. The person who lazily spends the entire day in an atmosphere of seventy, on a diet containing but little carbon, freely using ices and ice water, can hardly expect to feel vigorous and warm when he leaves his cosy corners for the open air of a cold winter's day. A diet of fat meats, sugar, molasses, buckwheat, with proportionate exercise, will enable a person to feel comfortably warm in a temperature of sixty degrees, thus greatly decreasing the difference between house and out-door temperature. But little additional clothing, on leaving his abode, will insure his bearing the rigor of a severely wintry day without discomfort. When this system, so much in harmony with the laws of nature, is pursued, colds, catarrh, rheumatism, neuralgia, bronchitis, pneumonia, and consumption, very seldom attack an individual. This being so with all, how much more so must it be with tender and sensitive girls from the ages of five to fifteen!

Girls who attend school, and remain motionless for several hours in over-heated rooms, are liable to constant derangements; and many of them perish before they are crowned with academical honors. Girls with a good circulation can sit as many hours in a temperature of sixty degrees without suffering; and when they leave that prison for the air of heaven, their lungs and skin will not be so easily impressed by the change of temperature. A brisk walk will bring roses to their cheeks, their system will re-act, and they will return home ready for a hearty repast.

Air, food, light, and exercise constitute the principal means by which the health of all human beings is maintained. Would that girls were allowed a sufficiency! Boys will get it anyhow, and it were well-nigh impossible to prevent them. But girls, subdued by training, and tied to the mother's apron-string, need the assistance and the authority of the physiologist in their cry for help. Oh, let the mother forget to lock the door, that her daughter may follow her natural instincts, and run for health in the air and sunlight of day, in the games and pleasures suitable to her age! The seraph of the household may become of a ruder complexion; her spirit, more buoyant, may encroach upon the stateliness of refinement; but what matter? Her mind, under this healthy *laisser-aller*, will grow strong in harmony with her body. Her stomach will digest; her heart throb with power; her sleep be undisturbed; her excretions normal; indeed, every organ will respond to the healthy regimen. Thus she will grow into womanhood prepared to fulfill her mission as nature intended.

On the other hand, imagine the fragile, narrow-chested, susceptible, delicate girl of the over-heated house, or of the narrow, badly ventilated apartment. A breath of cold air strikes to her very heart! Quiet, subdued, because deprived of vigor; susceptible to cold, because condemned to poor circulation of blood; sluggish in her functions, because of her general languor; having no appetite, because of want of wear and tear of her muscular system; nervous as a quivering leaf from want of tone; sleepless because unfatigued. This condition, so much in discord with the requirements of nature, can only bring forth the woman of tears—tears that will bathe every step of her course through life.

Were it not that our duty is imperative, we would have avoided the painting of this last picture; but, however painful to contemplate, it is presented in the earnest hope that the evils it delineates may be shunned.

CHAPTER II.

SOCIETY,

IN ITS RELATION TO THE HEALTH OF GIRLS.

A NUMBER of people living together in certain bonds of union, whether in tribes, in hamlets, towns or cities, constitute a community or a society. The very word *community* conveys the idea that the people composing it have objects in view that are common to all.

This is the crude principle that induces men to live in groups, forced into that position probably by the simple necessity of self-preservation.

Society may be defined as an improved condition of these groups, guided by the indefinite and unexpressed law of common consent.

One might live in a community unmolested and undisturbed, perhaps, simply by obeying the written common law, or abiding by the cardinal principle "do unto others as you would have others do unto you." Society, however, exacts more; it modifies or enlarges the scope of the law, without actually forcing any one into obedience, or administering physical punishment for non-acquiescence; still, these mandates, although not served with the official seal of the magistrate, are nevertheless compulsory, as another form of punishment—social ostracism—is sure to follow infractions. Moreover, compliance being optional in society, like a debt of honor, it is sooner observed than when forced by process of law.

All laws, to be suitable to a community, must be general, and cover the interests of many people, often spread over large space, as in states, nations or empires. They cannot, therefore, be so restricted as to meet the wants of closely united, although numerous, populations, which, in their turn, are sub-divided by occupations, industries and preferred modes of living. The society of Paris, as an example, might prosper under the general laws of France, but the variety of callings, professional and industrial, of its people require more; namely: rules and regulations governing the intercourse among its immediate members, that would be unnecessary and unsuitable to the much smaller groups sparsely located in agricultural districts. In short, cities need municipal laws.

The social system of law, unwritten and not subject to forcible compliance, is elastic, and therefore in the condition to be easily modified whenever circumstances or events require it, thus forming a complement to the written law of the land.

It is an important complement too; for without it the amenities, the good manners, and the refinement of large aggregations of people, would be lost in the simple observance of *meum et tuum*, the common law. Therefore, although much may be said against the unphilosophical and even unreasonable decrees that have gradually crept into the codes of social ethics, the necessity of some social code must be recognized.

Social customs, so often beneficial to well organized communities, may as often prove dangerous if yielded to without discretion or discrimination. Mushrooms growing in the bark of a tree may appear to the careless observer as an integral part of the same; but a little discretion will show the error. The mushrooms that grow on the diseased spots of social constitutions may appear the same and be respected accordingly; but a little examination will show that they are only unhealthy outgrowths, which should not be tolerated if the integrity of society is to be maintained.

Spencer, the erudite and searching philosopher, has analyzed these social fungous growths, and it is well worth while to read his works on sociology, for nothing is more interesting than his examination of social structures. But, here, we can notice only the errors which are honored more through custom or force of habit than for any good influence they bear on the health of the human economy. Fashion constitutes one of its departments, probably the most dictatorial, the most potent and irrepressible; its exactions, like all imperiousness, being as much for evil as for good.

In the varied departments of social government, fashion is probably the one that plays the most active part in the physical welfare of the people, and consequently it is a subject that cannot be overlooked in a guide to health.

Napoleon III., as a financial statesman, might at first sight have been deemed right in encouraging extravagance in his Court. The magnificent and varied costumes of Eugénie created a *furore* in the female community of the wealthy class for certain fabrics, certain colors and shapes of courtly robes. The silk manufactories of Lyons vied with one another in quickly supplying the market with the extraordinary requisitions; thousands of mechanics and laborers were kept at the loom and the spinning-wheel, and thus thousands were employed who otherwise would have been idle, troublesome, grumbling people. But, on the other hand, the extravagance of that court, becoming contagious, spread beyond the limits of the classes able to bear the enormous tax. The desire to be in the fashion contaminated all ranks, and extended beyond the boundaries of the nation for which it was intended. That extravagance filled many a coffer with gold; and for a while even the national exchequer was buoyant. But, like all unhealthy things, the disease unnoticed corroded the very foundations of society, and threatened it with general destruction. The panacea invented by the Emperor was one sure to fail. The sad episode of that country's trial in its war with Prussia, proved that the potion was only an alluring one; for weakness instead of strength had grown under its administration and in the passage-at-arms to which France was forced she was overwhelmed and conquered.

Eugénie, the Empress, plump and warm, might order transparent materials that her exquisite throat and well moulded arms be not entirely hidden; or some other Eugénie, lean and anæmic, but wealthy, might properly order heavy silk to cover her ropy throat and sinewy limbs. Eugénie in the Tuilleries, in gilded coaches and on velvet carpets, may adorn herself as is fitted to her position, and to her condition in life; but Eugénie, the wife of a humble citizen in moderate circumstances, with household duties to perform, may perish in the attempt to follow the Empress.

Eugénie of the Court of France may have a corset

artistically applied to her form, but Eugénie the wife of a city attorney may not have the famous artist at hand, and the corset bought at the store, although called "the empress," prove to be of inelastic material and totally unsuited to the form of the attorney's wife. Again, should Eugénie lose her natural hair, the imperial crown may not sit well on her stately head, and a competent artist may be called upon to supply the deficiency—but is that a reason why all women should adopt the fashion of wearing false hair? Yet this is done to-day, even by the kitchen maid; and where human hair is unattainable on account of costliness or otherwise, horse-hair and wool and all sorts of abominable imitations, in the shape of "rats" and "mice," are employed.

With the Empress dethroned, however, fashion's reign does not cease, for the manufacturers are still engaged in enticing its devotees. Trade is their profession, consumption the corner-stone of their palatial structures; but, as consumption *per se* would not be sufficient to enable them to gild the seat of their easy-chairs, variety and change must be continual, that gold may come by scattering abroad the flimsy products of their brain. These manufacturers employ no physiologist or moralist, but only the skillful artificer, who is expected to overshadow his old devices by improvising novel ones, thus making the blind followers of fashion the dupes and victims of the inventions of these gold mongers.

Reason, whenever at variance with fashion, is abandoned. Witness the ridiculous costumes, the induced deformities, the unnatural gaits, the transparent pretensions of respectable women who daily defy good sense in our public thoroughfares.

But fashion is found not only in dress. Let a foolish spendthrift of high rank invent a beverage or a flavored dish, and his boon companions will leave his halls impressed with the necessity for adopting it. Thus coffee and tea were imported from their indigenous regions, and, however unreasonably, have become articles of diet common to every culinary establishment. Unphilosophical minds argue that such articles could not be favorably received and generally adopted unless they were pleasing to the senses and innocuous to life. They little know how this pet theory of theirs would fail upon examination! Tea and coffee have done more injury to nations and to people to whom they are not suited, by reason of climate or temperament, than all the battles of the twenty years' wars of the great Napoleon. Physicians every day meet the victims of these drugs who have not even the Hotel des Invalides to repair to. They are not armless, neither do they walk upon stumps, but they are crippled in their whole nervous organization. Neuralgia, that most painful of all diseases, is so common to-day that a shrug of the shoulders is given at any one complaining of that infirmity. Coffee is the generative parent of that disease. Palpitations and functional diseases of the heart are common, too, to-day; tea should properly legitimate this offspring. That undefined affection misnamed "nervousness" should be more properly baptized under the name of "coffee-ism" or "tea-ism," and just as deservedly as the unbridled passion that engenders murder or the ill-treatment of a wife or the overthrow of the intellect is called "alcoholism."

Fashion becomes custom, custom becomes habit, and under their dominion man is but an abject slave.

Coffee, tea, or alcohol should not be denounced any more than the gunpowder that forces projectiles into millions of hearts. Their agency is well known and established; and if education would teach that powder is not to be used except for blasting rocks, alcohol for chemical and manufacturing purposes, and tea and coffee as medicines for those who need such drugs, their disastrous effects would cease and they be written among the list of blessings.

Educate the young not to follow baneful fashion, that injurious habits may not be acquired, and, above all, spare your children the effort of not imitating *you*, if devoted to it, and the coming generation will abound in health and beauty.

Exaggerations and misapplications of fashion are oftentimes not only dangerous, but absurd. A hat is an article of dress intended to protect the head, but ornamentation has often got the better of its usefulness. Woman's hat has been subjected to strange metamorphoses. As a bonnet it has been seen to look like an exaggerated coal-scuttle, hiding not only the hair, but a great part of the face. It was an ugly contrivance, but had some claim to usefulness, as it gave protection from the rain or the sun. As a hat, we have seen it no larger than a full-blown rose, hanging as a mere ornament from the hair. We may see it adorning such pretty faces that we are glad it is small; for a delicate, oval face, with bright eyes, a classical little nose, and pretty lips, so pronounced by the tiny hat coquettishly placed on the head, is surely attractive. But again, let us see the same tiny hat, with bright ribbons and gay flowers, on the head of a woman whose age it would be uncharitable to mention, whose face had attained the fullness of the moon, and a nose that gives unmistakeable evidence of having seen better days. The same little hat is there, but the face, though similarly prominent, is not the same in effect, and the coquettish little trifle becomes a monstrosity. So, fashion may prove a failure in ornamentation as well as in usefulness and healthiness.

If the inventors of fashions were people who studied the laws of health as diligently as they do those that govern Beauty, Art, and Money, humanity would suffer less, and even this book need not have been written. The long skirt, trailed through dust and mud, may be a source of revenue to the manufacturer, but is one of loss of health to the consumer. The hoop that spread the skirts in a wide circle around the woman may have opened a new industry, but it has favored the introduction of cold air upon the person that has chilled the limbs of many. The change that afterwards brought the skirt to fit tightly around the person may have secured another class of industry—bustle-making—but it has thrown an impediment in the way of locomotion that badly affects the wearer's comfort, and sometimes by badly adjusted pressure at the back induces great pain and positive injury. The elegant garter that the Countess of Salisbury dropped, and which gave rise to the *bon mot* of "*Honi soit qui mal y pense*," may have been honored by that royal salutation of King Edward and made immortal, but the pressure of like articles has caused the withering of limbs that otherwise would have had development and grace.

Much has been written of the pernicious influence of fashion, yet the most judicious advice in this regard has failed to elicit much attention from those who, desiring to please, would adopt anything by it suggested, however inconsistent with the laws of health. It is to be regretted that the desire to please is inculcated in the young sooner than the observance of natural laws and the refining influence of good taste.

Into what terrible errors has fashionable dress led woman, requiring her to be sometimes dressed, sometimes semi-nude! How catarrh, rheumatism, pleurisy, neuralgia, and consumption have reveled among the devotees of these conventionalities!

There was a time when woman dressed according to seasons, and the change was made in strict accordance with the almanac, for it was considered not *comme-il-faut* to do otherwise; and if the heavens respected the almanac less, it was the fault of the heavens and not of fashion, even if woman had to pay with her life for her conscientious observance. It should be said, however, to the credit of the women of the present day, that the continued remonstrances of hygienists have not been entirely unheeded, and that they exhibit in some things more practical sense than their grandmothers. Placing the skirts on the hips is certainly a salutary improvement upon the habit of fastening them above the abdomen and under the armpits; and in like manner the women of our day are more likely to look at the sky than at the almanac before dressing.

In olden times it was not uncommon, also, for women to lace tightly during the night that the bosom be kept high and shapely. It is to be hoped that this pernicious habit has disappeared.

The high heels of the last century, remarkable only

for inconvenience, threw the body forward, thus cheating nature of the provision that the body should rest upon the heel rather than upon the toes. That heel caused many a curvature of the spine and other deformities dangerous to child-bearing, and its brief re-introduction a year or so since was marked in its evil influence on such troubles.

Again, society in its complex demands has changed the order of nature. Night is for rest; for the Shadow is the inviting host that all animals obey. But society has decreed differently; light for work, shadow for pleasure. And it is therefore that the youth who has worked all day is met in the small hours of night, over-fatigued and oppressed, wending his way to the couch that has waited long to give him rest and refreshment. The girl, too, who has begun to relish the dangerous enticements of gay life—witness the *abandon* with which she will pass through the varied charms of an evening devoted to mad pursuit of "pleasure," and then go out into the inclemency of a winter night in a dress of "airy nothingness" to return to her home. The inspiring scenes of the ball-room having passed away, she helplessly sinks into a chair, to be relieved by her maid of the vestments that only force can remove. The removal of her shoes extorts an expression of pain; and when her corset, wet and chilled, is taken off, her body is variegated with the creases from its pressure. She now draws a breath such as she has not drawn for hours, and her lungs, heart, and liver are glad to be again set free. The imagery of the evening's excitement floating in her brain forbids sleep. If she arises next morning it is a wonder; if she has no headache it is a miracle! Haggard and pale she presents a very picture of debility.

Rest has hardly brought back the flush to her cheeks before a perfumed note is placed in her hand requesting the pleasure of her company to a similar *entretien du beau monde*. And so, night after night, until body and brain wilt in the dry heat of passion. This is homage to fashion; this is effort to please!

The exaggerations of fashion, injurious as they are to people of all ages, are particularly so to girls during the period of development. In some countries girls are kept in close confinement until they arrive at the nubile age; but while their minds may thus remain free from the taint of sensualism, impressed by too early contact with the world, their bodies must languish under restrictions that deprive them of physical exercise. The body and the mind should be allowed to grow apace, untrammeled by unnecessary restrictions or unseasonable stimulation. The education of the Convent may enhance the purity of the soul and refine the brain with intellectual power, but its efforts will be futile if the body, through which only that power can be exhibited, is undeveloped or diseased. This country, a very cradle of liberty and intelligence, errs in a contrary manner. Here, girls, who should only breathe the purer atmosphere of home, are allowed to frequent theatres, balls, dress like women of consequence, and share in all the allurements of society. Like premature flowers, they are forced into this unnatural life, exhausting their vitality long before they have secured the physical strength adequate to bear so much drain upon their nervous organization; hence the severe but just criticism, that "the beautiful women of

America do not last." Physically they are tired, morally they are wearied, until often at the age of thirty they are old in their faces and satiated in their senses. Having exhausted all in the nature of pleasure or fashion, in their *ennui* they might join in the lament of the renowned Georges Sand, who says: "In the course of my life, unrestrained either by rule or by rein, I have done as others. I have appeased hunger by savory and exciting nutriment. I have cheated sleep by a reveille without purpose or by unprofitable work. Sometimes by the light of my candle I have sought in books the key to the great enigma of human life; sometimes, borne by the whirlwind of the times, I have stood among the multitude with a sad heart and looked with somber gaze upon all the elements of satiety. In vain I have sought to seize in the perfumed air of nocturnal feasts, a sound, a breath, that would cause me an emotion. . . .

"High life, enervating to the organs and exciting to the mind, has closed the light of day from the palace of the rich, it has lit the torches to give light to wakefulness, and imposed the work of life upon the hours nature has marked for rest. . . .

"How resist this feverish race! How run in this breathless course without exhausting one's self before reaching one-half of the distance marked by the stake!

"So here I am, as old as though I were a thousand years. My beauty, so much praised, is but a deceiving mask, under which is written exhaustion of the body and agony of the heart. In the age when feeling should be keenest, I have no feeling, not even a desire, unless it were to end this life of fatigue and disenchantment for the repose of the grave!"

Thus speaks this woman, who has drained the cup of pleasure and excitement, ere she has run one-half of the cycle allotted to her life. In the whirlpool of gratification she has drowned even ambition, and she is ready to die.

To preserve the life of woman, to render her strong and capable of fulfilling her destiny, should be the purpose of the physician and of every man privileged to call her mother or wife. These two words, that fall from the lips of every being, from the cradle to the couch of death, may appear trivial on account of their constant use, but a complete order of creation is contained therein. If a mother were a mother but an hour, if a wife were a wife but a day, what comfort, what happiness would humanity enjoy? All that contributes to man's happiness is directly or indirectly from her, in her relative positions of wife and mother. What are children without a mother, what is home without the wife? Her sickness paralyzes the household; her death leaves a vacancy that cannot be filled. Wealth would be but a meaningless word were she not there to share it; ambition but a thorn were she not there to soothe and encourage; disappointment, or affliction, but fatal stabs, were she not there to apply the balm of hope and fortitude. The gray bearded man returns to drop tears of sorrow on the lap of his octogenarian mother. The trembling hand that smooths his rugged brow removes the sting of worldly injustice, and releases the victim from the clutch of passion.

Woman's part and lot in life is a grand one; no loud and discordant clatter of dispute about her "sphere" can ever give her higher, broader, or nobler duties and privileges than she has, as mother and educator of her race. Her position may be improved, legally, industrially, socially, by more enlightened enactments; and God speed that day! But meantime, and always, she will have in her own hand the key to greater power, and without it all reforms will be nugatory. She must seek, find, and keep her *bodily health*. Let the mother guard her daughter's footsteps, then, when she begins to enter on the perilous approaches to the realm and reign of Fashion. Society is full of pitfalls for the unwary, and its requirements often induce habits and practices which are found to be dangerous only by their evil effects. Then it is too late!

CHAPTER III.

EXERCISE,

IN ITS RELATION TO BODILY FUNCTIONS.

PHYSICAL exercise, systematically and judiciously taken, is the greatest harmonizer of the bodily functions. Muscular action induces destruction of tissue; should it go on without intermission of rest, and resupply of nutrient material to make good the loss, exhaustion would be the consequence. The loss of tissue creates a demand for nutrient elements, which is made known by the sensation called "appetite." Under this action and reaction, loss and supply, the integrity of the muscular and nervous tissue is maintained. The bones, too, brought into action by the muscles, receiving their quota of stimulation during exercise, grow, and develop into proper proportions. When exercise is partial, or local, the parts thus brought into activity grow out of proportion to the surrounding parts; thus the blacksmith exhibits a powerful and sinewy arm; the dancer a powerful and well developed leg. Exercise, therefore, when general, serves to develop in adequate proportions the various parts of the body, and, when partial, to strengthen those requiring better development.

Exercise quickens the circulation of the blood; the lungs, responding to the rapid flow, require a greater quantity of air for oxygenation; hence respiration is quickened to obtain the supply. The blood thus becomes purified in the lungs, and returns more rapidly to the tissues with new material for nutrition. The carbonic acid is thus quickly exchanged for the vitalizing principle, oxygen, that stimulates and gives vigor to the body. The pulse responds to this general tone, and consequently beats firmer and with a more even rhythm.

The union of oxygen with the carbon of the blood evolves heat. When the circulation is rapid, the carbonized blood reaches the lungs quicker, requiring a greater amount of air for oxidation; hence respiration is increased, and a greater evolution of heat is the result. Exercise, then, performs the triple function of assisting in the elimination of effete matter, of conveying more nourishment to the exhausted tissues, and of generating heat.

Long-continued exercise, uninterrupted by periodical and adequate rest, would cause exhaustion, as is evinced by the sensation of fatigue. This sensation is the warning that the time has come when a supply of nutritive materials should go to replace the waste of tissue already incurred. To secure a perfect distribution of the nutrient elements, rest is necessary; consequently exercise immediately after taking food is hurtful, as activity destroys so much of the nervous force needed for a proper performance of digestion.

Those who do not conform to these demands become dyspeptics, from non-assimilation of food

Excessive fatigue indicates a great loss of tissue, and is dangerous, because the system, under its general prostration, would not manifest its wants; and, while it may require food, it may not induce the sensation of hunger suggestive of such necessity, and therefore go unsupplied at a critical moment. And, again, if much food is taken when the stomach is weak from continued fatigue and want of nourishment, it may remain unacted on, and unassimilated, and become a source of irritation instead of force.

Persons leading a sedentary life, or a life of little activity, as shop-keepers, who would eat out of proportion to the wear and tear of their bodies, accumulate fat, become obese and lethargic. Hard-working men, on the other hand (and particularly students, who use up an immense quantity of nervous matter), unless properly and adequately supplied by rest and nourishment, would become very lean, and be the victims of neuralgic and pulmonary complaints.

Exercise, to be beneficial, should be proportionate to the strength, and have relation to the habits and occupation of the individual. Purely physical labor induces stupidity, and lethargy of the intellectual faculties. Purely mental labor reduces the volume of the body, and causes a debility that renders one prone to receive impressions from the slightest irritating casualty.

Society, intent upon refining girls by close application to study, neglects that fundamental principle of health consisting of the proper equilibrium between mind and body.

What is proper exercise for girls? Such a question, on a subject apparently so simple, need occasion no surprise; because custom, habit and fashion have so misdirected young women in this regard that they scarcely would understand now what healthy exercise means. In society, as constituted, girls have but limited opportunities for it.

MODES OF EXERCISE: WALKING.

A daily walk should be enjoined upon all girls, from infancy upwards, without paying too much regard to slight inclemency of weather. If civilization has done anything, it has certainly invented appliances for the protection from cold, from rain, from wind, and from the sun. The walk should be a pleasurable one if possible, and of sufficient length to induce moderate fatigue.

Walking is the first and most natural mode of exercise. The act of walking brings into play all the muscles of the body, and even the internal viscera partake of the general movement from the shock incurred every time that the foot touches the ground. The circulation and the respiration are accelerated in proportion to the exertion undergone. The senses are not passive, for every object attracts the eye and causes a thought. The changes of situation—as the being in the shade, under the sun, facing the breeze, quickening the step in the cold, slackening it in the heat, exchanging salutations with friends, or analyzing objects of curiosity—give an exercise of the organs of intellect as well as of the body which secures moral and physical equilibrium. It is therefore good for the sound in health, for the convalescent, and for the valetudinarian.

It is said that a systematic walker never dies of consumption. However true this may be, certain it is that those who form and carry out the resolution to take a daily walk generally enjoy good health.

RIDING.

Riding is one of the most enjoyable and salutary exercises known. This mode of motion is peculiar and ever-changing, and not dependent on the will. To maintain equilibrium, the rider must conform to the gait and the motion of the horse, which depend on the condition of the ground and on its own speed. Under this exercise the circulation and respiration are greatly increased and digestion assisted; the mind is pleasantly engaged, emotions excited, and emulation inspired. Young people like to ride well—some desire to exhibit prowess and skill. In many diseases riding is found to be more efficacious than the most renowned therapeutic agents.

Riding, in increasing the tone of the muscular fibers, in promoting digestion and assimilation, corrects morbid sensibilities, and is therefore of great benefit in hysteria, hypochondria, chronic neuralgia, palpitation from dyspepsia, etc.

DANCING.

Dancing is probably the most welcome, and certainly a most useful exercise for girls, though the difficulty is in getting it under proper conditions. It is a system of motions, composed, as an author has said, of running, walking, and jumping. It has been practiced from ancient times, although of late it has undergone serious modification. The dance of the ancients was an inspiration, that had but little form or rhythm. Civilization, more exacting in propriety, as society understands it, has checked the impulsive and ingenuous motions of the "inspired" dancer, to reduce it to an even, regular motion, that is fatiguing and tedious from its continued sameness. Waltzing has been introduced, which, in its rhythmical turnings can only weary the limbs, send blood to the head, cause dizziness and sickness of the stomach; it deprives the lungs of air, causing oppression from want of breath. Quadrilles, now almost entirely proscribed from the *salon* of fashion, are really a most excellent practice of gymnastics, particularly for girls of lymphatic temperament.

Dancing requires plenty of fresh and pure air to satisfy the greater circulation of blood in the lungs. The inspiring of a great quantity of air, surcharged with carbonic acid emitted from either burning gas or candles, and from the lungs of a multitude of persons present in a close room, is exceedingly dangerous. The motions occasioned by the various dances require that the muscles, and particularly those of the thorax, be free from the stricture of tight dressing.

Dancing contributes to physical education and development. It is a corrective of that sedentary life which keeps the lower extremities inactive; it is a pleasurable exercise, favoring sociability, and stimulating the desire for suppleness and grace; but care should be taken that the enjoyment of this mode of exercise be had only where the air is pure, and not over-heated; when the dancers may be properly dressed, without compression, or exposure to sudden changes of temperature; and in company and at hours which are wholesome both to the *morale* and the *physique*.

On this score, Michel Levi says: "The moral and physical influence of dancing is a therapeutical resource that promotes menstruation when late, or corrects many of its irregularities. On the other hand, when too often repeated, or carried to excess, it may excite the organs of circulation, so susceptible in a young girl, and cause reactions which are distinguished by debility, pallor, and languor."

ROWING.

This mode of exercise, for a specific purpose, namely, the development of a narrow chest, is one that cannot be surpassed. Under the alternate and continued extension and contraction of the muscles of the arms and of the chest, the ribs are kept in active motion, favoring, through this elasticity, expansion of the lungs. The circulation and respiration are greatly accelerated, thus adding to the exercise of those organs. The pleasurable excitement is conducive to a happy state of the mind. The air on the surface of the water is pure and invigorating. The motion of the body is graceful, and under these vitalizing agencies, girls of delicate respiratory or digestive organs will improve in health and strength, and acquire forms that are attractive in woman.

GAMES.

Billiards, so little practiced by woman, is one that stands pre-eminent among all games for healthful exercise. The constant change of attitude, the moderate force required, and the pleasure it inspires, fit it as the woman's game *par excellence*. Croquet, tossing ball, battledore, are games, which, being played in the open air, and moderate in their requirement of force, are also conducive to the health of girls.

PASSIVE EXERCISE.

Driving is a passive exercise which is healthful on account of the change of air experienced in the distance passed over. Driving to the country is far preferable to driving in the confined air of a city. The motion of the carriage communicates some motion to the body, which, although limited, exercises the muscles and the articular surfaces.

It is a pleasurable mode of exercise, and a great relief from continued and confining occupation.

Sea going. The sea air, the novelty of the situation, and, often, sea-sickness, prove salutary. Many invalids have found health at sea. The air is invigorating; it contains ozone, and the emanations of sea-salts. Sea-sickness deters persons from going to sea; but, really, it is seldom that it affects one in a distressing manner. The great majority of sea-going people feel the inconvenience for two or three days; after this they begin to feel better, and finally become perfectly well, enjoying an excellent appetite. The rest of the journey is passed without illness, and the general health is greatly improved. When nausea is present, the smells of the ship, which come from the stagnant water in the bilge, or from the oil used on the machinery, greatly aggravate the case and add to the discomfort. It is therefore well that persons apprehensive of sea-sickness should engage berths well-ventilated and distant from the engines.

Many are the hygienic expedients recommended to avert sea-sickness; but their comparative failure is only further proof of the general fact that things beneficial or curative to one are not so to another.

Some adopt the system of lying down as soon as they go on board, and remain quietly in their berths for several days, until they feel no longer that terrible *malaise*. Others will remain constantly on deck in the open air.

Both these methods are good, but the choice must be made from the experience of every individual; for that which will suit one may not suit another.

Passengers should go on board in good condition, at least so far as the biliary organs are concerned. The intestines should have been previously unloaded, even by a discreet purging. On board, for the three or four first days, food should be taken often, but in small quantities. Champagne, brandy, lemon juice, or pounded ice often relieves inclination to nausea, and even an intense attack of it.

Persons easily affected by the ship's motion should secure a position as near the centre of it as possible, as there motion is least. Keeping the perpendicular by swinging the body in the opposite direction to the motion of the boat lessens its bad effect.

Sea traveling often cures chronic diarrhœa of long standing, invigorates the biliary apparatus, and relieves biliousness. Hepatic, renal colics, and dysentery are also often cured. It is said that choleraic patients do well at sea.

SINGING.

This is also a mode of exercise about which little has been said regarding its effect upon the health of girls. A great hygienist, however, speaks as follows: "At the age when the system has not attained sufficient development, the exercise of singing is not without accident. In the natural state, respiration is divided in two equal actions, viz.: that of inspiration and that of expiration. In singing, the alternation is not regular or uniform; the inspiration by which the voice is sustained is held for a long time; the blood, unable to enter the contracted lungs, dilates the cavities of the heart, the larger veins and the capillaries; it is then that the veins of the neck swell and the face becomes red. It is thought that this suspension of a regular breathing tends to induce diseases of the heart and of the lungs, at least in delicate girls. Many girls, who are preparing for professional singing, have to abandon it on account of pulmonary hemorrhages."

It is therefore necessary to use proper judgment in this regard, and not force the practice of this art upon girls whose organization cannot bear the effort without suffering. Singing is an attractive accomplishment, but the health and life of a girl are of greater importance, and she should not be led into the practice unless her physical development warrants it.

Girls whose efforts to reach a high note are such as to make the bystanders tremble for fear of accident, should not sing. "A beautiful voice adds new charms to beauty, but the study of an art of pleasure should not be one of pain and danger."

It is principally for girls who attend school that exercise of divers kinds is imperative. Mental work and bodily inertia lead to nervous exhaustion and deformity. Gymnastics, adapted to their physical condition, should be practiced during the hours of rest. The importance of this fact is so generally known now, that all well conducted schools are supplied with proper gymnastic apparatus.

Exercise secures good digestion, maintains a good circulation, a proper temperature, and gives vigor to the body; it is therefore one of the greatest protectors a young woman can have.

CHAPTER IV.

FOOD,

IN ITS RELATION TO THE PRESERVATION OF LIFE.

THE selection of food should be based upon certain physiological and fundamental principles which ought to be understood by all and complied with as far as practicable.

Food has two great offices to perform: to maintain the natural heat of the body and to repair the waste of the tissues. In the young it has to supply extra material for growth. Without the first, the temperature of the body would fall below the standard consistent with the progression of life; without the second, the body would be self-consumed.

Speculative physiologists have calculated that one twenty-fourth part of the constituents of the body is changed in the course of twenty-four hours. This may seem very surprising; for the inference would be that a person weighing 150 pounds would daily require six pounds and four ounces of actual nutritive material; and, as it is further calculated that an adult excretes forty ounces of solids and fluids, it would seem as if nine pounds of food (solid and fluid) should be taken into the body within twenty-four hours to maintain its integrity. But all the nutrient materials are not taken in by the mouth; the skin absorbs some from the vapors of the atmosphere: hence an exact calculation is impossible. The skin is a very active agent, not only in secreting fluid for its own elasticity and in maintaining an equilibrium of temperature, but in absorbing life-giving properties. It is related of a jockey, who had been starved in order to be reduced to the proper weight for riding, that, just before taking his ride, he complained of great weakness and thirst; a cup of tea was administered, and in an incredibly short time his weight had increased six pounds, and he was consequently disqualified for riding. The warm cup of tea stimulated the skin into action, and every pore was opened to absorb nourishment from the vapors of the atmosphere.

This is another good argument in favor of keeping the skin free from impurities, else absorption would be prevented. It is impossible to give an exact estimate of the amount of nutritious material a person might usually take in twenty-four hours; as the amount required depends on the wear and tear of his system from labor, on atmospheric conditions, and on evaporation, etc. This uncertainty is, however, provided for by nature, in a proper system of balance. A slight excess would be relieved by excretions from the kidneys, by the sudoriferous glands, and by the lungs; moreover, another part of the surplus would be stored away in deposits of fat, as is usually seen in persons who eat more nitrogenous and carbonaceous food than the waste from the actual exercise of the body would require.

All food taken into the mouth is subjected first to a thorough mastication, and the action of the saliva; the saliva not only adding the water necessary to a thorough mixing of the substance under the triturating process of the teeth, but converting its starch into sugar.

In this operation the saliva secreted by a hearty and well-fed man has been estimated to be as high as three pounds a day, although Carpenter does not place his estimate higher than twenty ounces. Thus mixed and masticated, the food descends into the stomach, where the chemical action of the gastric juice and the mechanical action of the muscular fibres resolve it into an homogeneous semi-fluid mass, called *chyme*. The chyme passes onward through the lower orifice of the stomach (the pylorous) into the duodenum (the first portion of the small intestines, so-called from being of twelve fingers' breadth.) In the duodenum the chyme is mixed with the *bile* from the liver, and the *pancreatic juice* of the pancreas (the sweetbread, a gland of considerable size lying just below the stomach). These two last fluids chemically modify still further the new chyme, until it is reduced to a fit condition for absorption by the lacteal vessels, which, like a net-work, surround the whole intestinal canal. These vessels converge to, and end in, one common duct, called the Thoracic, which empties itself into the left jugular vein.

In the duodenum the chyme undergoes an important alteration, both as to its sensible and its chemical properties. The effect of the admixture of the bile and the pancreatic juice is to separate the chyme into three distinct parts; two parts may be said to contain the oily substance, the proteine compounds, the saccharine and saline matters in solution, constituting a compound emulsion called *chyle*, ready for absorption; and one, the residue, composed of insoluble materials and biliary matters, which, being unfit for nutriment, pass on into the intestines. and are finally evacuated as effete matter.

Careful observers have calculated the amount of gastric, pancreatic juice, and bile secreted by each respective organ in this work of digestion and assimilation; and it is given that a healthy man secretes in twenty-four hours thirty-seven pounds of gastric juice, ten pounds of pancreatic, and three or four pounds of bile. These quantities, as Hinton says, seem amazing, and if true they can only be explained by the supposition that they are quickly re-absorbed, and "that the total quantity may express the result of a rapid circulation, the amount present in the stomach at any one time not exceeding a few ounces."

The process of digestion had been a mere speculation of physiologists until Dr. Beaumont, of the United States Army, had a remarkable opportunity for witnessing it within the human stomach. It was the wound of Alexis St. Martin, of Canada, which, having left a permanent fistulous aperture in his stomach, enabled that clever physician to make those important observations which, afterwards, were confirmed by Blondot and Bernard, by similar experiments on dogs.

After many observations, Dr. Beaumont was enabled to determine the relative digestibility of the most important articles of diet. This was a valuable research, worthy of great consideration; for upon the digestibility of food greatly depends the well-being of all mankind, and particularly of persons afflicted with weak digestion, occasioned by constitutional debility. Almost any food might, in time, be digested by a healthy stomach; but the length of time required to digest separate articles of diet varies in different individuals. The knowledge of the digestibility of each article is of great service, because the longer an article of food remains in the stomach, the greater the work imposed upon that organ, which would eventually become exhausted in the repeated and continued attempts to reduce the indigestible materials.

The normal functions of the stomach may be affected by the quantity eaten, the nature and amount of exercise taken before eating, the length of interval allowed between meals, the general state of health, the condition of the mind, the seasons, the climate, &c. But a general knowledge of the digestibility of food, when the system is in good condition, may enable even the diseased to discriminate properly, and select the food that, on account of easy digestibility, may prove beneficial. Dr. Beaumont found that indigestible substances, when present in the stomach, interfere with the process of assimilation of the whole, and prevent an early reduction of the various articles taken at one meal into that homogeneous mass called chyme. According to his observations beef is more easily reduced than mutton, and mutton sooner than veal, or pork; fowls, when young, being less digestible than was supposed, and turkey more so than any meat except venison. He also ascertained that soup and fluid diet, so often resorted to by the sick, on the supposition of easy digestibility, are not so easily chymified as solid aliment; and this latter fact is often experienced by dyspeptic persons.

Dr. Beaumont's experiments confirm our notion regarding the effect of temperature on digestion, *i.e.*, that the free use of ice-water during meals, and ice-creams at dessert, is detrimental to the process of digestion. On one occasion, he observed that the injection of only a gill of water at 50° into the stomach sufficed to lower its temperature below 30°, and that its natural temperature was not restored for more than half an hour. The cooling of the stomach, at a time when it needs its greatest activity, must be injurious, and, in our opinion, is responsible for the majority of the cases of dyspepsia in this country, where cooling beverages are unsparingly used at repasts. It has already been stated that cold contracts the capillaries and drives the blood from them; deprive an organ of its circulation and you deprive it of its force; how, then, can a stomach perform its functions under the treatment of ice?

The use of ice-water at the table is an acquired habit, not a necessity, for we find that in the warm climates of Italy and Spain, ice-water is scarcely ever used; and the laboring classes of those countries, exposed to the heat of the sun, and warmed by actual exertion, find ice a luxury that they cannot afford; but they are the people who never suffer from dyspepsia.

Sherbets and ice-creams are luxuries delightful in warm seasons; but they should *be taken after digestion is completed*, when the stomach has no labor to perform.

Liebig has divided food into two principal classes: one, that he calls "*respiratory*," supplying the principles that are burnt, as it were, by the oxygen of the inspired air, to heat the body; the other, "*plastic*," supplying the elements to form tissues.

This division, although subject to criticism, may be accepted for its simplicity, the objections to it being only of such a nature as would confuse rather than aid the layman in comprehending the process of alimentation.

The food contributing fuel to the respiratory organs chemically contains large portions of carbon and hydrogen; plastic food, much nitrogen, and traces of phosphoric acid, lime, soda, potash, iron, magnesia, &c.

The elements of respiratory food are carried by the blood to the lungs to be exposed to the atmospheric air, the oxygen of which combines with them to produce carbonic acid and water. The chemical combination of the carbon and hydrogen of the blood, with the oxygen of the atmosphere, evolve heat and vapor; the heat warms the blood, thus keeping it to its natural temperature, and the water is exhaled by the lungs in a state of vapor.

A proof of the latter may be had, on a cold day, by blowing on a piece of glass, when the vapor will be condensed by the colder external air and form drops of water on the surface of the glass. The cooler the air, the greater the loss of heat from the body; it is then, therefore, that oil, fat meat, and all articles containing much carbon, are needed. An example of this we have in the diet of the Esquimaux and Laplanders of the Arctic regions, which often consists of the blubber of the whale.

Before experimental science had demonstrated that chemistry entered largely into the vital process of growth, separation of tissue, evolution of heat, &c., mankind followed in the track of all animals, and selected food by instinct; and it may be that instinct proved more salutary, for it was the voice of nature, and the food then selected was simple and unmixed. As the savages do now the whole human family did then, namely, gather food in its natural state wherever found.

But, in the course of time, populations greatly increased in number, and commenced to collect in localities, and formed aggregations of people for whom nature had not provided. It would be appalling to see three million Londoners start early in the morning for the fields and waters of England in quest of food! Cultivation of food and the exchange of one article for another then became a necessity, else those who were stationed in arid lands would have starved. While this semi-civilized state progressed it was found that wheat might be raised in certain regions, while fruits would grow better in others; that where land was too poor for cultivation water might yield its fish, animals be caught in the wilds, birds brought down from the air. A fish or a bird might then be exchanged for a loaf of bread, and so *ad infinitum*, until all could partake of the bounties of the earth. This is barter, or commerce in its incipient and natural state. But these communities had other necessities. While people tilled the land they could not make bricks nor build dwellings; they could not manufacture cloth, nor make clothing, &c., hence the exchange enlarged in scope, and gained in proportions, until the whole work of civilized humanity became divided in classes, each one contributing to the other.

But in bartering a difficulty arose: a man could not give a cow for a pair of boots, for it cost more time and labor to raise the cow than to make the boots. An equivalent was necessary, a medium that could balance the difference on a fair principle of equity. From this necessity money was invented, which having received a value recognized by all, and divisible into the smallest possible amounts, could be used to supply the deficiency, and thus enable persons to consummate an exchange between articles of different value. Thus multitudes became organized under the common law of equity. Society became a complex but perfect machinery, in the combination of which reciprocity was the motive power.

In this great combination of labor, for it is nothing else, the need of food is the motive power that impels humanity. Let food be scarce or unattainable and the frame of the social fabric will fall as if struck by a thunderbolt. That cohesive force once removed society falls asunder; each man following the crude instinct of self-preservation. Murder and rapine would be the ruling passions, and the civilization of a thousand years would disappear, as if by magic, from the face of the earth.

As these groups of population grew more numerous, and concentrated in fixed localities, such as towns, cities, &c., the demand for food increased in adequate proportions, and man sought it everywhere and in everything. Natural food becoming scarce, he was compelled to eat things he would never have eaten in his savage state; he studied combinations that should make things palatable that otherwise would be repulsive; he has added condiments and cooking, and finally made of the *cuisine* an art that is almost a science. But in all these praiseworthy endeavors the love of money has prevailed even over natural necessities; and articles unfit for food have been invented, carefully prepared and introduced, until now it is very questionable whether the man who partakes of the repast of the wealthy is not worse off than the poor laborer whose limited means compel him to still live on the simple productions of the earth, prepared in a primitive manner. It is questionable, too, whether the common law of equity, born of the above mentioned necessities, has been fairly carried out; for it is evident that in bartering some persons get the better of others, and are thus enabled to accumulate wealth; that is, the means to provide themselves with luxuries by shrewdness rather than by labor, while others have yet to work to earn every loaf of bread,—although we must acknowledge that brain-labor may be more than the equivalent of hand-labor, and skill in labor of any kind will always be worth more (that is, will produce more) than mere unintelligent force. It is questionable also, whether the accumulation of wealth has contributed much to the well-being of the accumulator; for we generally find better health and more contentment among the working-classes than amongst the opulent. It is particularly of *health* that we speak, for we are conscious that the pleasures of the table have done more work of death among its devotees than all the battles of the savages in their struggle for existence.

As civilization has advanced, however, men have devoted themselves not only to the production of food but to the study of its quality in relation to the health of the human economy. They became learned in the science of anatomy and physiology, and speculated on the natural functions that reduced all articles taken as food to a condition to be assimilated, and distributed to the system for its preservation. We shall not attempt to follow them in their exhaustive disquisitions, but hope to be able to draw a sketch of this wonderful process of nature, that will awaken the interest of the reader, and induce further search in abler and more elaborate works.

The circulation of the blood carries the nutrient materials to the source of life. Life is constant until it ceases forever; so the circulation of the blood must be constant. Hours of rest are not periods of intermission but only of less activity. At the very moment that the heart ceases to beat life is extinct. We would compare the circulation of the blood to water running a mill. By way of illustration, let us suppose a mill, run by water flowing through a canal of a circular form. It may be said that this is admitting an impossibility, for a circle cannot have a constant declivity, without which the water would find its level and come to rest. But let us suppose it, nevertheless, because the figure may be easily conceived by the mind. That water, kept in motion by force, would go round the canal circle and strike the paddles of the mill-wheel and make it turn. In doing this, however, the water would be constantly exposed to loss of quantity from evaporation and from absorption by the soil. It would then constantly decrease in quantity until, at a certain time, it would become so reduced as not to be sufficient to propel the paddles of the wheel, and the mill would come to a stop. What is the remedy? To keep the mill constantly to its work water must be supplied to the canal in proportion to the loss. So with the circulation of the blood. The blood is the fluid that carries supply and force; lessen the supply (the nourishment) you lessen the force until the heart stops and death ensues. But in the human system the blood is more important than the water is to the mill, for the blood not only conveys force, but the supply to replace the material used up in the work of the human machine, which is not the case with the water; and the mill, consuming itself by its own work, will last only for a time proportionate to the consumption and the ravages of moisture and heat. The blood, on the other hand, carries the supplies for the maintenance and the integrity of the organization, supplies the oils for lubrication, the fuel for a normal temperature, absorbs the residues of used and useless matter, carries them to the filtering organs, and thus keeps itself pure and ready to absorb constantly the life-giving elements of food.

If this were not true it would be a charming fiction; but it is true, and is a wonderful evidence of the wisdom and design of the Creator.

We must quarrel with the so-called "rationalists" or "naturalists" for their attempt to choke our admiration with their dictum that all this is the work of Nature, that even a blade of grass is organized on the same principle. Allow it. What then? They have only changed one word for another. They worship at the shrine of Nature; we, at the shrine of God. They can not explain their Nature any better than we can explain our God. Both may be abstractions, but the conception of a God is the conception of a *personal power*, which, however infinite and omnipotent, is not an idea impossible to human understanding; while Nature is an abstraction without a comprehensive unit, a mist on the imagination, an impenetrable cloud in the firmament of our intellect.

Were nature merely a chemical combination, capable not only of analysis, but synthesis, it could be reproduced by chemistry at the hand of man. But all the analysis that man has been able to make of nature has been only proximate, never intimate; hence, although the chemist may ascertain by analysis the properties and proportions of the elements of certain substances, say, wood, for example, he can not take those elements and produce wood by any chemical process. Why? There evidently is a something that his analysis has not discovered. What is it? The vital force belonging to the organic kingdom. The body of man has been analyzed, nay, all the elements of his composition have been discovered and carefully weighed; yet the chemical philosopher cannot make a hair, much less a human body. Even as regards food, he knows all the elements composing it, yet pure chemical elements could not maintain the life of the body. Oxygen, hydrogen, nitrogen, carbon, and even the salts, are trophies of chemical art and science, but avail nothing to the body in their chemical purity; they must be in an organized state to be useful to it. There is something, then, in that *organization* which the scientist cannot reach, else we could receive our food from the chemist instead of from the butcher and the grocer. All that enters the body, ere it becomes a part of it, must acquire the properties of life and be modified by the vital force of the body, not by chemical principles; it must conform to the rules of *organized* life.

It must not be supposed that inorganic matter acts within the body as it does in the retort of the chemist; the elements must obey another law than the chemical, —*the law of vital force*. All the glands and cells of the various organs have their duty to perform,—to reduce all the elements, simple or compound, absorbed or taken in to peculiar conditions acceptable to the primitive organization. This duty cannot be performed by art or science.

The transformation of the articles of food within the body is remarkable. Solids become fluids and fluids become solids. They must become fluid to pass through the thin membranes of the vessels and pass out of the same; they become solids in the bones, the muscles, the nerves, the hair, the nails, &c.; again they become fluid to be filtered by the kidneys, and even gases to be exhaled by the lungs. Does chemistry do this? No; vital force does it. What is vital force, then? Here we ponder; philosophers give no answer.

But vital force is exercised in the body at the expense of the tissues, just as much as the work of a pulley is at the expense of the rope. This consumption would be a disintegration of the tissues, unless vitalized food went to replace the loss. Particles devitalized by use are of no avail, and are therefore cast off by the same vital power, through the kidneys, the skin, the lungs, the intestines, &c. All materials of the body that have become useless to the organized structure are expelled, and from that moment cease to be a part of vital organization and are turned over to their original master, chemistry.

It is thus that all excretions soon give signs of decomposition; for, deprived of the maintenance of vital force, the elements separate in obedience to chemical laws, and in the process gases are evolved that are offensive to the sense of smell.

The circle of life is as follows: the heart (the left chamber) propels pure blood through the arteries into all parts of the body; the tissues take from it the new material and give up to it the worn and useless; as the blood takes up the waste it becomes impure and returns through the veins to the opposite chamber of the heart (the right); in its course thither it takes up the new elements of food that have been prepared in the stomach and are poured in through the left jugular vein by the thoracic duct, as above explained. The venous blood, charged with impurities and the elements of new food, is now propelled by the right chamber of the heart over the surface of every air-cell in the lungs; the oxygen of the atmosphere passes through the air-cells and oxydizes or burns out the carbon, the most noxious element of the impure blood. The union of the oxygen with the carbon creates carbonic acid gas, which is exhaled from the lungs at every expiration. The chemical union of those elements evolves heat, which maintains the proper temperature of the sanguinous fluid. Some of the hydrogen of the blood unites also with some of the oxygen of the inspired air, producing water, which also is exhaled from the lungs in the form of vapor. The blood, thus purified, returns to the left chamber of the heart to be propelled again to the tissues of the body. Thus the circle is complete and the flow of its vital fluid constant.

The work of purification is not all done by the lungs, however, for the venous blood on its route to the heart passes through various stations for purification; the kidneys take from it the urea and the salts of ammonia, the liver its bile, the skin other noxious fluids.

This work, although so briefly stated, is very complex and easily deranged by the quality of food. It is known how quickly a poison can disturb and even destroy it; it may then be easily comprehended how even slight but continued errors in diet may so derange it as to induce evil consequences.

A bad digestion is the source of countless evils. Not only the physical but the moral life is greatly affected by it. Passion, anger, irritability, hypochondria—all these malarial vapors arise from the black fountain of indigestion, and cast a wide shadow of sorrow and suffering which all who are unfortunate enough to come within its limits must share. The dyspeptic himself is the central figure of this unhappiness that radiates bitterness and pain towards all who approach it, not excepting even those who would assuage with love and tenderness. Physically he is a martyr condemned to administer to himself his own poison. Food he must have, though every mouthful becomes a flame of fire; for hours after he has taken it he is on the racking wheel, and relief comes to him only when the food has passed away.

Let young people ponder all this; let them commence early to shun indulgence in eating and drinking; let them understand the part that digestion plays in human life; for if they practice prudence they will preserve stores of happiness that will help them in every struggle; make them youthful in old age, though their limbs are withered and decrepitude steals over their bodies. Youth is the father of old age; the seeds that are sown when young will bear fruit when old.

Three things must be understood in the selection of food: materials for producing heat, materials for replacing waste, and materials to supply growth.

"The want of material to keep the muscles, organs and tissues from wasting will cause the sensation of *hunger;*

"The want of material to supply loss of brain or nervous tissue—*mental sluggishness* and *nervous debility;*

"The want of material to supply the lungs with fuel, sensation of *cold;*

"The want of fluid to supply the loss of water in the body, sensation of *thirst.*

"The blacksmith who hammers his iron, the carpenter who planes his board, use muscle almost exclusively. Some of the muscle is constantly consumed and eliminated by perspiration and urination. Should they continue their muscular labor without tarrying to repair the loss by a hearty meal of muscle-making material, they would soon fall exhausted to the earth.

"The student in his cell, consuming brain-element in the solution of mental problems, while the muscles are in a state of quiescence, would soon become insane or idiotic, should he not rest to repair the loss by a meal of brain and nerve-making material.

"A walker, consuming muscular element and throwing off a great deal of water in perspiration, would soon become as stiff as a board, should he not rest to eat, and to drink water to maintain the suppleness of his muscles.

"If man, in the exercise of his physical or mental strength, needs a supply equal to the loss, the child will need a supply adequate to its growth. Moreover, a child may be deficient in muscle, but precocious in mind; it may be lean, grow slowly, and yet show a high degree of mental activity. *Vice versa,* its muscular system may show a great development, and its mind very little power; in this case the child may be very fleshy, well developed, but stupid. A rickety child lacks bony matter, as is evinced by its inability to walk, and by the curving of its limbs when it stands. Again: a child who has no brain work to do, and spends its time in running and jumping, will require muscle-making material; while one at school, deeply engaged in its studies, will require a constant supply of brain-making element.

"In providing food for the young, therefore, the above suggestions should be borne in mind, so as to be able, as far as possible, to supply the proper proportions of the elements required. In cases where the system appears properly balanced, a diversity of articles can be taken at a meal to supply a reasonable quantity of the elements without disturbing the equilibrium. The appetite, which is the language of our need, is rightly satisfied only when just enough of each element has been taken to supply that need. If a person needs carbonates, he may eat nitrates in great quantity and yet not feel satisfied; and so *vice versa*, one needing nitrates would not feel his appetite satisfied by eating carbonates, even in excessive quantities." (Verdi's *Maternity*.)

The relative proportion of nitrates, carbonates, phosphates and water of various articles of food has been carefully noted by analytical chemists; and here will be appended a list of the most important articles thus analyzed, for the convenience of the reader—the figures showing the *percentage* of the elements named, in the articles analyzed:

FOOD.

	Nitrates.	Carbonates.	Phosphates.	Water.
VEGETABLE FOOD.	Muscle-Making.	Heat-Making.	Brain and Bone Making.	Waste.
Wheat	15.	69.	1.6	14.
Barley	17.	69.	3.5	14.
Oats	17.	66.	3.	13.
Northern Corn	12.	73.	1.	14.
Southern Corn	35.	45.	4.	14.
Buckwheat	8.	75.	1.8	14.
Rye	13.	71.	1.7	13.
Beans	24.	57.	3.5	14.
Peas	23.	60.	2.5	14.
Rice	6.	79.	.5	13.
Potatoes	1.	22.	.9	75.
Sweet Potatoes	1.	26.	2.9	67.
Apples	5.	10.	1.	84.
Milk of Cow	5.	8.	1.	86.
Human Milk	3.	7.	.5	89.
ANIMAL FOOD.				
Veal	16.	16.	4.5	62.
Beef	15.	30.	5.	50.
Lamb	11.	35.	3.5	50.
Mutton	12.	40.	3.5	44.
Pork	10.	50.	1.5	38.
Chicken	20.	35.	4.	73.
Eggs, White of	15.	none.	4.	80.
Eggs, Yolk of	17.	28.	5.	54.
Butter		All Carbonates.		

From this table, we infer that a *precocious* child should not be fed on *fish*, or such articles as abound in *phosphates*. But a child at school, and consuming brain material, would require that class of food; and if, besides, the child is lacking in muscular development, barley, oats, beef, etc., should be added.

"On a very cold day, when a child is to go out, buckwheat cakes and molasses would be an excellent preparatory diet, while it would be a highly improper one on a hot summer day.

"For a child who plays games, or runs, *nitrates* and *carbonates* would be required to keep him in strength and heat." (*Maternity*.)

Liebig, as we said before, divided food into two grand classes; the *respiratory*, or heat-producers: the *nitrogenized* or tissue-making.

To the first class, he has admitted all FARINACEOUS, SACCHARINE and OLEAGINOUS substances. The farinaceous includes the cereals, such as wheat, barley, rye, oats, maize or Indian corn; the pulses, as peas, beans and lentils; the pith of trees, as sago; the roots, as arrow-root, tapioca, potatoes, etc.; these articles contain starch, which becomes converted by the saliva into sugar—sugar being chemically composed of carbon (charcoal) and water.

The *saccharine* embraces grape-sugar, honey, cane-sugar, figs, dates, prunes, beets, mangoes, carrots, turnips, etc., which differ but little from starchy substances, namely in the greater proportion of water.

The *oleaginous* is derived both from the vegetable and animal kingdom, as fat, lard, animal oil, butter, seal and whale oil, and the olive, linseed, walnut, and other nut-oils; these containing a great proportion of carbon, nitrogen, and but little water.

On the above division life could be maintained in its integrity as is commonly done in some agricultural districts where animal food is not largely accessible.

The *nitrogenized* or *albuminous* class is derived from the animal as well as the vegetable kingdoms, and particularly from seeds, as peas and beans, from eggs, the flesh of animals, fish, milk and cheese.

The *gluten*, the gelatine of animals and various salts are also good articles of diet, but only when mixed with the above two classes.

The *sub-acid fruit*s are also contributors to healthy food; their laxative properties assisting in relieving bulk from the intestines, such as apples, pears, plums, apricots, peaches, cherries, strawberries, nectarines, melons, pineapples, and oranges.

The *digestibility* of food has also been an object of great interest to the physiologist. Spallanzani, Gosse, Tiedman, Gmelin, Sir Astley Cooper, Trousseau, Lallemand, and many others of more recent date, have sought by innumerable ways to discover the difference between the various articles of food in the time that each required to be digested. But it is due to Dr. Beaumont to say that his careful observations and experiments on the human being are preferable to the results obtained by other physiologists from their experiments on dumb animals.

The opening in a human stomach gave Dr. Beaumont great advantage over other physiologists, but this fact renders his discoveries only the more reliable. The labor of these men has not been in vain; for although they differ in some immaterial points, their differences are quite consistent, inasmuch as digestion is in some degree dependent upon age, sex, temperament, idiosyncracies, moral and physical condition, occupation, climate, etc., and as it is well-nigh impossible to find two persons exactly in the same condition, their powers of digestion may be different. From the experiments of Dr. Beaumont, Trousseau has gathered, first, that the meat of mammals is less easily digested than that of birds, and much less than that of fish; second, that they are all more digestible when roasted than when fried or boiled; third, that beef is more easily digested than mutton, mutton than pork, domestic fowl than wild, fresh fish than salted; fourth, that dishes prepared with milk are the most digestible of all except fish; boiled milk more than fresh, cream more than butter or cheese; fifth, that soups are not very digestible; but that farinaceous vegetables are, particularly when cooked. Fruits and green vegetables are also said to be easily digested.

Here below will be found Dr. Beaumont's list, arranged so as to show the time averaged by each article of food in undergoing and completing the process of digestion. They are placed in succession, the most digestible preceding the others:

ARTICLES REQUIRING NOT MORE THAN AN HOUR.

Boiled pig's feet, boiled tripe, boiled rice.

FROM ONE TO TWO HOURS.

Fresh eggs, beaten; salmon, boiled rye, broiled venison, broiled beef, liver, boiled milk, raw eggs, codfish, tapioca in soup, saur-kraut

FROM TWO TO THREE HOURS.

Fresh milk, fried eggs, roasted wild turkey, boiled wild turkey, roasted domestic turkey, roasted goose, broiled lamb, boiled gelatine, boiled beans, oysters, lean beef roasted, beefsteak, broiled mutton, salt pork, poached eggs, chicken broth, bean soup.

FROM THREE TO FOUR HOURS.

Boiled beef, broiled pork, roasted mutton, roasted oysters, boiled carrots, broiled sausages, dried beef, stewed or roasted; hard-boiled eggs or fried, mutton broth, oyster soup, melted butter, old cheese, wheat bread, broiled veal, domestic fowls, beef soup.

FROM FOUR TO FIVE HOURS.

Old salt beef, boiled; salt pork, fried or boiled; bone broth, fried veal, wild duck, boiled cabbage, roasted pork.

The same article is often found in more than one of the above lists, but it will be noticed that the manner of cooking is different, and that it is under the varied treatment that its digestibility becomes modified.

The experiments of Dr. Beaumont have been made upon one man, and should, therefore, be taken with some degree of allowance; yet it must not be forgotten that that man was in a state of general good health.

It is also well known that articles easily digested by one person prove very indigestible to another; and *vice versa;* yet there is a general fitness of things even in food, and the observations prove that Dr. Beaumont's experiments, although taken from one single individual, may serve as a safe and practical guide.

DOES FOOD AFFECT INDIVIDUAL CHARACTER?

Liebig observes that the carnivora are generally stronger, bolder and more pugnacious than the herbivorous animals on which they prey; and in like manner, those nations whose food is derived from the vegetable kingdom differ in disposition from those who take it from the animal. Houghton says: "The hunted deer will outrun the leopard in a fair open chase, because the force supplied to its muscles by the vegetable food is capable of being given out continuously for a long period of time; but in a sudden rush at a near distance, the leopard will infallibly overtake the deer, because its flesh-food stores up in the blood a reserve of force capable of being given out instantaneously in the form of exceedingly rapid muscular action." The horse and the dog might be similar examples; the swift greyhound may, in a spurt, advance beyond a swift horse, but the horse will beat the dog in the long run, although it may carry considerable weight on its back. Fothergill asserts, with other physiologists, that the energy of the British soldier is to be attributed to his liberal dietary of beef. M. Metz, of Mettary, the benefactor of the children in the Reformatories of France, declares that stubborn and refractory boys could be subdued by a vegetable diet, while the weak-minded could be made to hold to their resolutions by a generous diet of meats and wine.

Absolute rules for diet are impossible, yet one which should never be infringed is *moderation*. The gratification of a *moderate* desire is seldom hurtful; the stomach has a language of its own, and its demands seldom deceive. But persons who have abused the stomach with indulgence, or by habits that are not in conformity with the preservation of a normal digestion, may have cravings which it would be dangerous to gratify. The alcoholic drinker craves stimulants, yet the application of stimulant is only a means to encourage an evil that has become a disease, and that will hasten disorganization and death. Gourmands and drinkers should take care how they gratify the cravings of a diseased stomach. In this case only a skillful physician is competent to advise the regimen.

Girls, generally less active than boys, need not so much nitrogenous food. Their exercise being less, they require less tissue-making food. At the age of puberty, however, and on account of their loss of blood, more nutrient food may be required to supply the deficiency.

In treating of the diseases peculiar to women, the diet appropriate to each case will be suggested.

The golden rule should be in all cases, *Eat to live ; do not live to eat*. Eat slowly and *masticate* thoroughly. Preserve your teeth by keeping them clean, and not subjecting them to injury by sudden change from a high to a low temperature, or *vice versa*. This would crack the enamel and expose the spongy bone inside of it to the corrosion of acid, and the destructive effect of the air. Every defective tooth should be protected with a filling by a skillful dentist, or be extracted.

At meals the mind should not be preoccupied by cares or sorrows. This has been understood for so long, that the ancient Greeks and Romans at meals sought delectation in music and the comicalities of clowns.

Never take very active exercise, or sleep, immediately after a heavy repast (sleep retarding circulation); the stomach needs blood and quiet for a good digestion.

Do not cool your stomach with ice, sherbets or ice creams after a meal.

Do not eat to satiety; better rise with a feeling that you might eat more, than as if you could not give place to another mouthful.

Eat at stated hours; our system is the creature of habits; irregular habits are baneful.

Do not go too long without eating; a too long interval without food, particularly if at work, will debilitate the stomach, and disable it from digesting when food is taken.

Animal food is heating and exciting; vegetable, cooling and soothing; meat makes more blood, but requires longer time to digest and needs more bodily exercise, else it will induce plethora.

As animal food increases the circulation, the activity of the organs, and the heat of the body, it should be sparingly used by persons of sanguine and bilious temperament, of excitable disposition, and by those liable to inflammation and hemorrhages. It will be more suitable to temperaments of a lymphatic character, cold, indolent and phlegmatic.

Meat swells less, produces less gas and is therefore useful to persons liable to flatulence.

It is with some hesitation that we lay down this chapter, knowing how much the welfare of man depends on proper diet; yet we cannot go further without entering into such details as would increase its volume beyond the scope of this book. We cannot but trust, however, that the hints herein given will be of sufficient interest to make the mind crave for more, as the literature on this subject is by no means scanty.

CHAPTER V.

CLOTHING;

ITS LESSONS IN THE PRESERVATION OF THE LIFE OF GIRLS.

NATURE, so bountiful in every provision for the protection of life, has scarcely ever demonstrated greater wisdom than in the selection of coverings for animals that inhabit regions of the earth of different temperatures. Man, however, who is not limited to either space or latitude, she has left naked, but endowed him with an intellect capable of selecting such covering as season or locality may require. By these means he is enabled to migrate from one part of the world to another, exposing himself to violent atmospheric changes without danger. Food and respiration, although great contributors to the maintenance of bodily heat, would not suffice in the glacial regions, where the loss of caloric is above what nourishment and oxygen can provide. Had man been provided by nature with a permanent covering, it is easy to conceive that he could not pass from an arctic to an antarctic region without exposing himself to such sudden shocks to his constitution as would imperil his life. It is true that the natural covering of animals undergoes necessary modifications in conformity with the changes of seasons, and often of climate; but never so far as to enable the white bear of the glaciers to live comfortably at the tropics. Some animals, however, migratory by nature, select the climate best adapted to their nature; but those are they which are endowed with great swiftness of locomotion, as certain birds, and with the power to fly a thousand miles without rest in a comparatively short time; moreover, this is possible only to those whose food is easily obtained from the air, from the earth, or from the water.

The habits of man, and all his necessities for existence, are such as to localize him. He cultivates the earth that it may yield him food, and in such quantity as will provide for him against the uncertain future; he stays by his stores, and therefore does not feel compelled to leave the place of his birth in search of supplies.

Every surface radiates heat, and man, to prevent such radiation as would lower the temperature of his body below the standard consistent with the preservation of its existence, envelops it in clothing. The amount of radiation of caloric from the body depends also upon the condition and the temperature of the air immediately surrounding it; and as these conditions are many, in the different parts of the globe, and changeable even in the same locality, according to seasons, it follows that the materials for clothing must vary in their power of retaining or radiating heat. He has, therefore, taken from the animal kingdom, skins, furs, feathers, silk, wool, etc.; and from the vegetable, cotton, linen, jute, etc.; their adaptability for dress depending upon their power of conducting or retaining heat.

All articles of dress are more or less bad conductors of heat, and are interposed between the external air and the surface of the body as mediums to adjust, at all times and under all circumstances, the proper proportion of radiation and absorption of heat compatible with the integrity of the body. The very limited stratum of air which, however, is left to fill the place between the clothing and the skin, and also within the interstices of the material itself, is warmed by the radiation from the body and remains so, protected by the outer clothing, maintaining thus next to the skin a medium the temperature of which is neither too high nor too low; for the same power that the material has to prevent the quick transmission of heat from the body to the outer air it has to prevent the transmission of heat from the atmosphere to the body. Experience has practically demonstrated that a cover that will keep a body warm in a cold temperature will also keep it cool in a heated one.

The radiating or absorbing power of the material depends upon its color, its quality, texture and shape. Black absorbs, white reflects, caloric rays. Ice exposed to the rays of the sun will melt quicker under a black than under a white cloth.

Heat-conducting power is very feeble in wool, silk, fur, feathers, and all materials, in fact, derived from the animal kingdom; hence they are used in the winter season, and in northern latitudes. The intelligent and economical housekeeper surrounds her ice with flannel to prevent its melting rapidly, just as she envelops her babe in blankets to keep it warm, wool being a bad conductor of heat. Linen, flax and cotton, and all clothing material from the vegetable kingdom, are better conductors of heat, and are therefore useful in the summer season, and in regions where the temperature is generally elevated.

The various materials for dress have also electrical relations; silk, wool, fur, and feathers possessing in a high degree the power, not only of developing but of retaining electricity; while flax, linen, and cotton are good conductors, and diffuse electricity. It is on account of the above-stated facts that rheumatism, neuralgia, and all nervous diseases that are benefited by the electric current, are ameliorated by wearing silk, wool, or fur, while they are aggravated by linen, or cotton.

The shape of clothing has also to do with the maintenance or loss of heat of the body. A cover drawn tightly around the limbs, not permitting a stratum of air to be interposed between the cloth and the skin, would necessarily be cooler than a looser garment that would allow some air in the space between, for air is a bad conductor, and the clothing serves as a shield from the outer air that would otherwise absorb the heat from the enclosed stratum. The intelligent gardener, without much knowledge of science, protects his tender plants from the frost on the same principle, namely, by spreading a cover over them, which stops radiation, the natural cooling process.

The Roman flowing robe for women and the toga for men were probably the most physiological vestments for that climate, leaving the limbs free to act, and yet preventing radiation sufficiently to keep the body comfortably warm. In latitudes where the thermometer falls below zero, such open dressing would allow too much exchange of air, and the stratum above mentioned could not retain the degree of heat necessary to health and comfort. In spite of fashion, however, intelligent communities have, upon experience, settled on a width of garment which is best adapted to the atmospheric conditions as well as to the different occupations in life.

The only article of woman's clothing which attracts

the attention of the physiologist, on account of the objectionable tightness, is the *corset*. This article of dress is of comparatively modern invention, having been introduced by Catherine of Medici. Bouvier, who has given attention to the modes of dressing the chests of women at various periods, says: "Anciently the women wore chest-bands. In the first century of the French monarchy, and during a greater part of the Middle Ages, they vacillated between the Roman band and the new invention, *the body to the dress; i.e.*, the robe cut in two, the upper, called the *body*, fitting closely around the chest, while the lower part is left as a flowing skirt, a dress that prevails to this day. Towards the end of the Middle Ages the latter had prevailed. After the sixteenth century, corsets, stiffened with whale-bones, were introduced, which, modified to some extent, have continued to the present day." So much has been said about this article that it would seem but a work of supererogation to say more; yet it is a subject of such great importance that even with the danger of running into repetition, it will be here again noticed.

While it may be said that it is a support to the breasts, that it affords comfort to the wearer, it may be answered that a simple band, appropriately applied, would do as much; that all women do not need such a support, and that it is in this very instance where it is most injurious.

The corset, as adopted in modern times, is a stiff, unwieldy instrument, covering tightly a large and most important part of the body. It is kept in place by its own pressure, which is exerted over the muscles of the chest, over the cavity of the stomach and of the abdomen, thus reducing their natural capacity. When pressing upon the bosom, it prevents its development, and sinks the nipple into its substance, rendering the process of nursing almost impossible; pressing upon the chest it prevents a full expansion of the lungs by its fixed limits, and by paralyzing the muscles; pressing on the abdomen, it retards the circulation of the blood so important to the organs contained therein, it reduces the cavity and forces the intestines downwards, the latter pressing the womb, which eventually becomes the victim of displacements; pressing upon the stomach, it reduces its capacity and its power of muscular motion, necessary to the process of digestion. That article of dress therefore may, when used only for the purpose of vanity, be the source of dyspepsia, consumption, prolapsus and ulceration of the womb, leucorrhœa, constipation, and hemorrhoids, so common among the most fashionable class of women.

As to the relations of *color* to dress, it is, for our purposes, chiefly a matter of heat. A cook wishing to heat water rapidly places it in a black caldron over the fire, or wishing to keep it warm for a long time after its removal from the fire, places it in a shining white pot. Experience has taught that; but the explanation is that black is a conductor of heat and that therefore when the heat is external it will pass more readily through a black caldron, and would as easily pass outwardly should the same black caldron be used to retain the fluid after the fire is withdrawn. White being a conductor of much less power would not heat the water so rapidly when exposed to the fire, but would retain the heat longer when the surrounding air is cooler than the water.

Dr. Stark, who has made experiments upon the heat-conducting power of color, has come to the conclusion that black stands first, blue second, red third, green fourth, yellow fifth, and white last.

Count Rumford and Sir Edward Home recommended that black be preferred in hot climates, in the shade (and, we suppose, when the external temperature, however warm, is below that of the body, namely, ninety-eight Fahrenheit) because the heat would more quickly radiate from the body. That is even said to be the reason why the negro is able to live in a hot atmosphere; for, although under the sun he would absorb more heat than the white man, in the shade he would also radiate more, and thus bring about the wonted compensation. The same authorities declare that colors differ in power of absorbing moisture, and that, in that connection, they follow the rule of their heat-conducting power, and therefore suggest that in miasmatic localities, and particularly after the sun has passed below the horizon, persons should wear clothing of light color in preference, and they even blame the physician, a person more exposed to contagion and infection than any other, for his preference for black in his articles of dress.

GENERALITIES.
REGARDING THE CLOTHING OF SPECIAL PARTS.

Head.—The head should be *kept cool*, particularly in children, as heat predisposes that organ to congestion. The adult need wear but what will protect from the rays of the sun and from the rain. Non-conductors, as felt, silk, wool or furs, are generally injurious. The loss of hair so common among men is from wearing around the head materials that retain both heat and moisture. In the countries where women wear but a veil upon the head, as in Italy, Corsica, and the East, the hair grows luxuriantly and does not fall. False hair and other appliances, used to give a fictitious volume, injure the growth of the natural hair on account of the weight they impose and the heat and moisture they retain.

The Neck.—The blood circulation of the neck is not only great but superficial, the carotid arteries and the jugular veins being near the surface. Pressure around the neck, therefore, would be highly injurious, as it would prevent the flux and reflux of blood to and from the brain. The use of furs around the neck, except in extremely cold climates, is mischievous, by inducing perspiration to which the air has easy access, cooling it rapidly, and thereby producing catarrhal diseases and sore throat.

The Trunk.—This part of the body, containing so many noble organs, requires the most intelligent treatment in the way of dress. In climates where the changes of temperature are sudden, flannel is the material that should surround it, for it retains heat and prevents a too quick evaporation. In climates of a more even and moderate temperature, cotton or linen may be worn with comfort, provided the person wearing the same be not exposed to drafts of air even on a hot day. The condition of persons should be taken into consideration at all times; for delicate persons of lymphatic temperament, evolving but little heat, or persons subject to catarrhs, bronchitis, pneumonia, rheumatism, and neuralgia, should wear flannel at all times, although its thickness may be changed in accordance with the temperature of the atmosphere. The partial exposure of the chest, so customary among women of all ages, is extremely dangerous, from the radiation of the natural heat of that part and the quick evaporation of its moisture—a cooling process which predisposes to congestion.

Extremities.—An old adage says, "Keep your head cool and your feet warm." Thick soles are great protectors to the feet; leather, being but a feeble conductor, keeps them cool when placed upon a warm soil, and warm when upon a cool one. The paper soles formerly so much used by fashionable women are injurious. Their thinness and elasticity cause the foot to yield to every unevenness of the ground, rendering walking so tiresome and painful as not to be prolonged without discomfort. Fortunately, Fashion has grown sensible, and now prescribes substantial soles for women to walk on.

Tight shoes punish the wearer with both corns and bunions, and therefore need but little discussion on our part;—fashion and vanity have done much to injure the feet of our women. A good shoe is a shoe that fits, it is neither too large nor too small; a large shoe injures by friction. High heels change the center of gravity of the body, throw the knees and pelvis forward, and the upper trunk backward to maintain equilibrium, thus predisposing to dangerous curvatures of the spine.

That consummate hygienist, Hufeland, laid down certain precepts about dressing that we gladly quote here:

"Dress should not prevent the evaporation of the body, and not be so heavy as to fatigue. Furs should be discarded, because they retain too much heat, excite perspiration, and prevent evaporation. In this case the deleterious matter given out by the skin is retained on the surface of the body, becomes absorbed and injurious to the organism. For this reason too warm clothing is injurious to feeble constitutions, and to persons subject to rheumatism. Young people in good health should adopt light vestments in preference to very heavy and warm ones. Exercise is the best producer of heat for young people and assists evaporation. Fat, pork, cheese, candies, are creators of heat, causing no evaporation, and, therefore, should be avoided, particularly during warm seasons.

"Persons who have passed the meridian of life, when animal heat and evaporation are on the decrease, should wear garments of wool; and those of a lymphatic temperament, inclined to fat and indolence, those leading a sedentary life, and those subject to catarrh, mucous discharges, diarrhœa, dysentery and gout, should be particular in observing this rule.

"Wool is also beneficial to persons subject to congestions, vertigo, neuralgia, ear-ache, rush of blood, cough, pain and oppression of the lungs. Wool excites the skin, relieves the blood by evaporation, and is therefore a preventive of consumption, hemorrhoids, and all bloody flux. It is useful to those whose nervous power is feeble, to hypochondriacs and hysterical persons. It is a protector against cold and heat, dampness and wind. It is preferable in latitudes where atmospheric changes are sudden and frequent. It is not beneficial to persons who perspire easily, or who are possessed of much electricity, nor to all those who have great vitality, or who are predisposed to cutaneous eruptions. *All clothing made of wool* should be *changed* often, because it retains the emanations from the skin which would become a source of irritation."

Ed. A. Parkes, military hygienist, also says: "Wool being a bad conductor of heat, and a great absorber of water (hygropic water) is superior to cotton or linen. During perspiration the evaporation from the surface of the body is necessary to reduce the heat which is generated by exercise. When the exercise is finished the evaporation still goes on, and to such an extent as to chill the former. When dry woolen clothing is put on after exertion the vapor from the surface of the body is condensed in the wool, and gives out again the large amount of heat which had become latent when the water was vaporized. Therefore a woolen covering, from this cause alone, at once feels warm when used during sweating. In the case of cotton and linen the perspiration passes through them and evaporates from the external surface without condensation, the radiation of heat then continues. These facts explain why dry woolen clothes are so useful after exertion."

Pettenkofer shows by experiment the absorbing powers of wool compared with linen, and comes to the same conclusion.

During convalescence, from debility and lack of red globules in the blood persons are very susceptible to cold; hence, flannel should be worn by them, particularly when the debility is a consequence of rheumatism, intestinal inflammation, and pulmonary diseases.

There exists a prejudice against wearing wool in the summer season; but that is due to the ignorance of the fact that the danger to health is from a too rapid evaporation of the fluid emanating from the skin. The laborer in hot countries always wears his flannel, knowing that otherwise he would be easily chilled. To demonstrate the cooling process of evaporation one has only to come out of a bath and remain undried for a few minutes; unless the air surrounding the body is of a very high temperature and moist, the person will become chilled in a very few seconds.

Governments have now discarded linen in the clothing of soldiers; and in Italy, in July and August, the soldier wears his woolen uniform, and at night, when exposed to malaria, while on duty, a white woolen cloak. (See suggestions about colors, p. 158.)

REFLECTIONS UPON DRESSING.

(From Author's "Maternity.")

"Dress is not intended to be simply a cover to our nakedness; it has been invented in civilized countries as a protection of the body from vicissitudes of weather, and sudden changes from a high to a low degree of atmospheric temperature. Dress is to maintain within the body a certain amount of heat required for the circulation of our blood, the action of our organs, muscles and limbs. We know the effect of extreme heat or extreme cold on the human body; hence we can easily imagine that even in the intermediate degrees they must produce effects which, although not instantly fatal, will nevertheless induce changes in our system incompatible with the laws of health.

"The object in dressing being to prevent this evaporation of necessary heat from the body, it follows that, according to the elevation or falling of the surrounding temperature, the dress must be adapted. Heat must be equal, evaporation must be equal. To maintain this equilibrium, the body must be *equally dressed all over*.

"As the temperature affects the circulation it follows also that when the dress is partial the temperature is unequal, and the circulation of course unequal also.

"From the moment the circulation is unequal the blood flows more freely in one part than in another. The part more exposed to evaporation, or to a lower degree of surrounding temperature, will have a circulation slower than the parts protected from both. The cooling of the surface induces contraction of the capillaries, which drives the blood away from them—making them very sluggish, to other parts—making them very active. From the moment this fact is established the equilibrium is disturbed, and the human machine deranged in its operations. The great study of keeping a clock in perfect running order is to maintain the equilibrium of forces amongst the different parts. When one part, like the pendulum, chain, spring, or wheel, is differently affected by the surrounding temperature the expansion becomes unequal, the equilibrium is lost, and the clock is out of order. Philosophical mechanics have discovered this, and have used every skillful means to balance the gains and losses in the expansion of the metals by using metals of equal susceptibility, or of such known variations that the changes of one are compensated by the changes in another, &c. If we are so careful with clocks, why are we not with ourselves?

"Civilization, with all its wonderful apparatus for heating houses, will have done a great injury to mankind unless it provides also the means to protect us when we leave our luxurious homes for that open temple where the sun is the only fire and its satellites the only luminaries in its absence.

"The transition from 70° Fahrenheit within our abodes to zero without, must be productive of sudden changes in our circulation, unless clothing prevent it by being equally and sufficiently spread over the entire body.

"The feet, that touch the ground, which, in its cooled state, would absorb much of their heat, need adequate protection, else the equilibrium will be disturbed and a cold be the consequence. The dress of women is not calculated to protect their lower limbs and the abdomen as well as the upper part of the body; this is another great and general source of disturbance of that equilibrium. Those former parts become sluggish in their functions, and finally the seat of permanent derangement; the bowels become costive, the womb subject to congestions, congestions inducing painful menstruation, leucorrhœa, prolapsus, ulceration, &c.

"The chest or thorax, if not equally protected all over will be liable to the same functional disturbance. The lungs, being thus subject to a flux and re-flux quite irregular, will become disorganized; coughs, sore throats, pleurisy, pneumonia, consumption, must follow. The heart, the recipient and propeller of the blood, must become deranged when this fluid is constantly varied in its flow. If more blood is driven to it from the surface of the body than its natural capacity can receive and propel, the heart must become enlarged and enfeebled; its delicate valves, that are to open or close according as the heart receives or expels, must become troubled and finally disorganized; and then we have a sad condition of things, which can only bespeak an early death or permanent invalidism. The liver, kidneys, &c., are subject to the same influences and same risks.

"As it is with partial exposure, so it is with tight lacing. Pressure drives the blood away from the parts, the veins and capillaries being intensely elastic. Pressure not only prevents development of the parts, but actually causes absorption of the tissue. Tie a leg sufficiently tight to prevent the circulation of the blood for any length of time, and it will dwindle into incredible smallness.

"Commence early, therefore, in the education of dress. It is beautiful to look on the dimpled arms, chest, and and legs of an infant; but think of the consequences! The idea that exposure makes them hardy is not bad but then expose all parts equally, and do not keep them for eighteen hours in a temperature of 70° and six hours in an atmosphere from 10° to zero.

"If custom forces you into these incongruities, see that your child goes out into the fresh air with a body equally covered. Bare legs and bare arms are not conducive to its hardihood where the other parts are heavily clad. Better it should go naked, like the savages, and that your houses had no fires. Pleasure-grounds and shady-sides have sent millions of little beings to untimely graves. It is not the fault of the pleasure-grounds nor the shady-sides; but it is sitting on the grass and on the earth of a temperature much lower than the body, when the clothes that come between serve only to cover it from sight, not to protect it from the absorption of its heat. If a child is lightly clad, spread a shawl or a cushion underneath; a grown person in the same condition would do the same; it is only those delicate little creatures that are allowed such careless treatment.

HOW DRESS MAY AFFECT GIRLS.

"We all love to see children looking pretty, cunning, and attractive. The vanity of mothers does a great deal towards the attainment of this aim. Let us commence from the period that a girl baby leaves off her long robes for short skirts. The mother will take care that the baby's chest is well covered; the pretty limbs, however, will be exposed, the little stockings short, and the drawers made of cotton or linen, but thin. If the child goes out: "Nurse, put a sacque on the baby, and do not let her go out without her hat, it is cool to-day!" Unless it is decided winter, no additional clothing is suggested for her limbs or abdomen. The child goes out, sits on the ground, the temperature of which being lower robs the child of some of the heat from the legs and the lower part of her body. So the child goes from year to year without much difference in her apparel, the dress of the lower half of the body being much less in proportion than the dress of the upper half. The putting on of an extra *skirt* does not help this difference a great deal. In a small child the skirts are so short that they cannot be considered sufficient to keep the child warm any better than an umbrella carried above one's head. The cold air must necessarily get under the skirts, and the warmer the body the quicker the air will rush up—on the principle of a flue.

"In this way the temperature of the body of the girl, from her waist down, is kept from year to year several degrees lower than that of her body from the waist upwards.

"*The consequence is serious in the extreme.* Every one knows that cold contracts the skin, veins, and arteries, and propels the blood from the surface. Put your hand in ice-water for a few minutes, and you will see it shrunk and colorless, for the blood has been driven from it. This process is going on all the time that the child is less warm in one part of the body than in another. In the coolest part the circulation becomes slower as the blood is driven away. Where is the blood driven to? To the other parts of the body, where it is not wanted, where it clogs up and actually causes passive congestion.

"What is the first ill effect produced? *Constipation.* The bowels, like the stomach, have their functions to perform in digestion; they require the same quantity of animal heat; they require unobstructed circulation.

"But to expose the surface of the abdomen causes great evaporation of needed heat; the cold drives the blood to the interior, causing a clogging up in the internal circulation; the digestion, robbed of the heat, its operation interfered with, becomes gradually slower, all its functions slower and delayed; and constipation is a natural result of the whole. Is this not true. Witness eight women out of ten constipated! Why are men not so prone to constipation? Because their dress is calculated to *keep the whole body of an equal temperature*, and their circulation unimpeded. Witness the children of the poorer class. They may be exposed as much, nay, a great deal more, than those of the wealthier class, but their exposure is not partial; if they are thinly dressed, they are so from head to foot; if they have no drawers, they have no flannel shirt; if they have no shoes they have no hat. Constipation, then, is the effect of unequal dressing.

"But, again, constipation is the almost *universal cause of displacements of the womb*. These congestions of the womb, inducing leucorrhœa and ulceration; these frequent retentions of the menses; this universal painful menstruation; these irregularities, depriving the woman of her health, her vigor, her happiness, are all due to this unequal dressing, which by causing unequal circulation implants the seeds of disease and disorder from earliest infancy.

"When will woman love her children better than fashion? When she does, when she dresses them according to physiological common sense, then, and then only, will our women be strong and healthy; then will they go without sick headaches and neuralgias; then will they go without constipation and piles; then will they go without the eternal "pain in the back."

"How can the mother secure this? As soon as the baby is old enough to wear short dresses, let the mother, according to the season of the year, dress her *equally all over*. If it is summer light drawers will do, as she will wear but little above. As the cold season comes on, and she puts on the baby a flannel shirt, let her put on her flannel drawers. If she thinks the child needs more for the protection of her chest, let her think that the child will need as much for the protection of her limbs and abdomen.

"Thus let this system be continued, not until the

girl has arrived at the age of puberty only, but even after, and until she will need no dress at all.

"How does constipation cause displacement? If the bowels are not moved daily, fecal matter must accumulate within, distend them, and finally deprive them of the natural elasticity that causes them to expel the obnoxious contents. When they get loaded they press downward and all around them; they press down the womb, or they impact the rectum, and thrust the womb forward upon the bladder. They press upon the arteries, and prevent the purified blood from going to give sustenance to other organs. They press upon veins, and prevent the return of blood, causing a clogging up of the hemorrhoidal veins, which, in their turn, cause "piles;" or of the veins of the limbs, causing "varicose veins." The veins, so distended, ooze out water from their walls, and cause dropsy. Thus constipation, together with the continual draft on the abdomen, will cause congestion of the womb; congestion will cause inflammation; inflammation will cause leucorrhœa and ulceration; and all these disorders will cause such debility of the womb as will disable it from carrying a child longer than six or eight weeks; hence the *constant miscarriages occurring*.

"Let the mother bear this in mind; let her save her child from constipation, and she will save her from a hundred and one disorders that will render her life a misery. And, to do this, let her begin with the child's *earliest years*, to dress her *equally all over*."

"THE COWL DOES NOT MAKE THE FRIAR."

This truism, we are almost inclined to say, is not true;

if not in its literal sense, at least in its philosophical acceptation. Dress is more often an outer expression of self than that saying would imply. There is disguise in everything; but we think the disguise is the exception, not the rule. If persons acting in a disorderly manner should be suddenly arrested by a person in the garb of a policeman, and receive from the latter the order to follow him to the nearest police-station, nine out of ten would follow without questioning his authority. If, in time of war, persons going on a certain route to a common destination should suddenly be halted by a man in the recognized uniform of a soldier and ordered to return, nine out of ten would return without asking for his commission. A needy person, out at elbows, unwashed and uncombed, found on one's premises, is at once looked upon as an intruder, or suspected as a robber, and probably thrust out unceremoniously. But if the person is neatly and comely dressed, the inquiry might be made of him in a polite manner, "What do you wish, sir?" The thief that wants to pick the pocket of a gentleman dresses himself in the conventional garb of a gentleman. It is true that in his case the dress does not make the gentleman; but his experience has taught him that in the majority of cases it does, and therefore he trusts that his exception will not be detected.

Clothes are emblematic. A neat, well-dressed person is generally a person of order; slovenly in his dress, he is most likely to be slovenly in his habits and in his thoughts.

A philosopher says: "All visible things are emblems; what thou seest is not there on its own account; strictly taken, is not there at all. Matter exists only spiritually and to represent some Idea and *body* it forth. Hence clothes, despicable as we think them, are so unspeakably important. The soldier even in citizen's dress bespeaks the soldier, for his coat is trim to his body and his breeches must fit his well-turned legs. The farmer, even in soldier's dress, is the farmer still; for buttons trouble him, and his easy going is interfered with by the close-fitting uniform; he lets it bag, and looks the sloven farmer." So the dress is the external expression of the body within. There are those who affect to despise the conventionalities regarding dress, but such persons suffer from a misconception of its true character.

Neatness, uniformity with conventionalities, without entering into the excesses of fashion, is at all times the most attractive element of dress.

CHAPTER VI.

AIR.

ATMOSPHERIC CONDITIONS IN RELATION TO HUMAN HEALTH.

HUMANITY dwells in a sea of air, as fish dwell in a sea of water; and as the latter must be affected by the quality of the water, so the former must be affected by the condition of the atmosphere. A study that would enable us to at once detect the multitudinous changes and varied conditions of the atmosphere would be not only useful but immense. Such a work is, of course, impossible in connection with this book. Yet feeling that the omission of a subject so pertinent to hygiene would in great measure defeat the object sought to be attained, the conditions of the atmosphere that more generally affect the human economy will be treated in this chapter, classified as follows: hot and dry—cold and dry—hot and moist—cold and moist; movement of the air—mountain air—sea air; rapid changes of temperature; impure air of dwellings; effect of combustion of coal, wood, gas, oil, candles, etc., on the air we breathe.

HOT AND DRY ATMOSPHERE.

Under the influence of this atmosphere the internal organs are debilitated, while the external ones are excited. According to Michel Levi, the skin is the first to undergo modifications; its color is heightened, the flux of fluids swells it, which is relieved by an abundant secretion, known as perspiration. When this fluid finds exit through the skin, the urine decreases and the internal mucous substances become dry, causing a sensation of thirst.

The elevation of external temperature tends to raise the temperature of the surface of the body in a higher degree than that of the organs of the interior. The rarefied air, containing in proportion less oxygen, causes the lungs to work harder for a sufficient supply; hence respiration is accelerated; the heart follows the same necessity for the purpose of oxydizing the blood already surcharged with carbon.

The capillaries are peculiarly excited by the flux of blood, and by the effort to relieve themselves of the pressure. Under this abnormal stimulating process and loss of water, the internal linings become dry, the appetite decreased, digestion languid, and intestinal action slow. The great loss of water to which the blood is subjected, and the rapidity of its course stimulated by dry heat, predisposes to that plethoric condition which induces congestive headache, sunstroke or apoplexy. Even when its effects are not serious or alarming, the head feels heavy, the mind oppressed, and a general lethargy, causing repugnance to motion or activity of any form, supervenes. The nervous system becomes prostrated without commensurate action, producing even the opposite effect of lethargy—namely, restlessness and insomnia. Persons having inhabited latitudes where hot and dry atmosphere prevails will undoubtedly concur in the above assertions.

COLD AND DRY ATMOSPHERE.

This atmosphere affects people according to individual

temperaments; the bilious-sanguine temperament being able to resist a cold and dry atmosphere better than a lymphatic. Age has also its influence, as old people and infants are less able to bear it. Food increases the ability to resist a low temperature, as it is well known that oily substances containing a large proportion of carbon supply that element to the body, which, when coming in contact with the oxygen inspired from the air, evolve the heat necessary for the maintenance of life. The Esquimaux, in conformity with this natural law, subsist on meats containing great proportions of oil, or even on oil itself.

The physiological effect of a dry and cold atmosphere is to contract the organs of the surface—namely, the skin and its capillaries—and thus determine blood to the interior, causing congestion of the organs therein situated; the heart becomes oppressed, general stagnation of the circulation is induced, which, when carried to excess, produce lethargy and general paralysis.

The effect of cold depends, however, upon the reacting power of the person exposed to it, as experience has taught that the power of resistance to cold is different in different individuals. But continued exposure to cold predisposes even the strong to inflammation of the bronchial tubes (bronchitis), of the substance of the lungs (pneumonia), of the muscular fibres, or of the synovial lining surfaces of the articulations (rheumatism). Hence these maladies are more frequent in winter than in summer, and are induced by suppressed capillary circulation; and in pulmonary affections also, by the excess of respiratory action in the attempt to hasten combustion for the production of necessary heat.

DAMP AND HOT AIR.

It is well known that this atmospherical condition favors decomposition of animal and vegetable matter, during which process gases injurious to health are evolved. It is a heavy atmosphere, that induces debility, disturbs the appetite, and renders all the functions of digestive organs slow. Under this pressure respiration is impeded, and the heart, thus oppressed, beats feebly. The body, absorbing moisture, becomes heavier, and the kidneys are forced to make extra efforts to relieve it of the excess of water, from which follows a greater secretion of urine. Evaporation of the surface is prevented by the surrounding moisture, and hence perspiration can not come to the relief of the sufferer.

Humidity is also an absorber and a good conductor of miasmas; so that in crowded cities, where malarias emanate from the filthy surface of the streets, endemics and epidemics are likely to prevail during warm and moist weather.

The effect of this atmosphere upon the nervous system is quite remarkable, as evinced by the melancholy, bad humor and weariness felt by some people who suffer while it prevails. "In chronic lung diseases moist air is generally most agreeable, as it allays cough. The evaporation from the lungs produced by a dry atmosphere appears to irritate them."—*Parkes.*

COLD AND HUMID AIR.

This atmosphere is generally dangerous to human life, because the water held in suspension is a conductor of heat. Persons exposed to it feel keenly its effects, heat being extracted from them very rapidly. The dampness deposited on the surface of the body is another source of abstraction of animal heat. One is more quickly chilled in a damp than in a dry, cold atmosphere. It is on account of these facts that the inhabitants of our Atlantic coast feel the cold more quickly when the thermometer is at 40 degrees than the people of Minnesota when their thermometer stands below zero. Cold dampness reduces the transpiration of the skin to its minimum without producing the tonic effects of dry cold air. Under its influence the tissues are relaxed, vitality is lowered, the circulation less active, and the respiration slow in decarbonizing blood; the evacuations of the kidneys and intestines increase, while digestion and appetite fail; rheumatism, catarrh, and scrofula abound where this atmosphere prevails.

Michel Levi, in relation to the effect of atmospheres on the human system, sums up as follows: "Electricity stimulates the nervous system; light affects the coloring and plastic elements of the blood; heat acts on the skin, excites the liver, and irritates the brain; cold favors hyperemia by increasing respiration, digestion, and nutrition; humidity affects the cellular tissue and the mucous membranes, and tends to increase the white fluids; dryness maintains the tone of muscular fibres, facilitates the evaporations of the skin, and induces harmony in nervous action."

MOVEMENT OF THE AIR.

Parkes says: "This is a very important climatic condition. The effect on the body is twofold. A cold wind abstracts heat, and, in proportion to its velocity, a hot wind carries away little heat by direct abstraction, but, if dry, increases evaporation, and in that way may in part counteract its own heating power. Both, probably, act on the structure of nerves of the skin, and on the contractility of the cutaneous vessels; and may thus influence the rate of evaporation, and possibly affect also other organs."

It is on account of the too quick evaporation of the body that sitting in a draft is so dangerous.

MOUNTAIN AIR.

"As a curative agent mountain air (that is, the consequences of lessened pressure chiefly) ranks very high in all anæmic affections from whatever cause (malaria, hemorrhage, digestive feebleness, even lead and mercury poisoning), and it would appear from Hermann Weber's observations that the existence of valvular heart disease is, if proper rules are observed, no contra-indication against the lower elevations (2,000 to 3,000 feet). Neuralgia, gout, and rheumatism are all benefited by high alpine positions. Scrofula and consumption have been long known to be rare among the dwellers on high lands, and the curative effect on these diseases of such places is also marked; but it is possible that the open air life which is led has an influence, as it is now known that great elevation is not necessary for the cure of phthisis." (Parkes.) Dr. James Blake, of California, a reliable authority on the treatment of phthisis, adopted the plan of keeping his patients in the open air, and recommended them to sleep out, even without any tent; the result, it is said, was an astonishing improvement in digestion and sanguinification. Our experience during the war corresponds with Dr. Blake's. Many soldiers who passed through Washington in the most precarious condition from pulmonary affections returned strong and in a perfect state of health; and upon inquiry they stated that in a few weeks after camping out, in tents or without, their digestion improved, which was followed by a quick and remarkable improvement of the whole system. They went out as invalids; they returned with vigor renewed and health restored.

SEA AIR.

By reason of atmospheric pressure more oxygen is absorbed by the same number of inspirations on the sea than on the mountains. The air is kept pure by the almost constant breezes and vapors containing saline properties, and is less hot in summer and less cold in winter. It is therefore very useful to lymphatic temperaments, to persons affected by chronic maladies, as scrofula, chlorosis, anæmia, neuralgia, dyspepsia, and hypochondria. It is peculiarly adapted to girls of late menstruation, affected by leucorrhœa, hysteria, general debility, or displacements of the uterus from the weakness of the suspensory ligaments.

The sea air of the temperate regions of Florida, South Carolina, or of the shores of the Mediterranean and on the western side of the Rocky Mountains, is of extreme value to invalids with lung troubles, particularly during winter.

Sea air acts as a tonic, increasing the appetite. The infinitesimal doses of iodine, chlorine, soda, and potassa contained therein greatly assist in the cure of scrofulous diseases, as tuberculous phthisis, glandular enlargements, chronic diarrhœa, &c.

RAPID CHANGES OF TEMPERATURE.

"The exact physiological effects of these rapid changes have not been traced out, and these sudden vicissitudes are often met by altered clothing or other means of varying the temperature of the body. The greatest influence of rapid changes of temperature appears to occur when the state of the body in some way coincides with or favors their action. Thus the sudden checking of the profuse perspiration by a cold wind produces catarrhs, inflammations, and neuralgia. I have been astonished, however, to find how well phthisical persons will bear great changes of temperature if they are not exposed to moving currents of air; and there can be little doubt that the wonderful balance of the system is soon readjusted." (Parkes.)

AIR OF DWELLINGS.

The health of the community and of every individual is proportionate to the purity of the air breathed. Everything added and foreign to the constituents of pure air will, when breathed, affect the human organism unfavorably. Considering how many impurities emanate from the earth, and particularly from localities crowded with animals or loaded with decomposing vegetable and animal matter, it is rarely, except on mountains and on the sea, that air chemically pure is found; it is therefore our duty, and particularly the duty of those who superintend the raising of tender children and girls of susceptible organization, to study and learn the modes and means by which pure air is rendered impure, so as to be able to secure for those under their care the air that is compatible with human health.

Impurities enter into the air in the form of vapors, gases, or solid particles. Oftentimes these impurities cannot be detected by taste, smell, or sight; and they are then more dangerous on account of being breathed in quantity without a knowledge of their presence. This fact should render people careful, and anxious to know the nature of these impurities in order to prevent or avoid them.

It must be borne in mind, as a cardinal principle, that every animal would be a nuisance unto itself unless means were adopted to get rid of the emanations of its body and the exhalations of its lungs.

The limit of the life of a person, placed in a room of a given size, but air-tight, could be very easily prognosticated by measuring the amount of air contained in the room. At every second he would consume its oxygen and taint it with carbonic acid. For instance, an adult exhales fifteen cubic feet of carbonic acid in twenty-four hours; when the proportion of carbonic acid has reached fifty to a thousand cubic feet of air, it has become fatal to human life; hence in a room of one thousand cubic feet, *i.e.*, a room say ten feet square and ten feet high, the person inhabiting that room would die in three days and three hours. This length of time is given, assuming that only carbonic acid would exist there as impurity; but his life would come sooner to an end on account of other impure emanations from his skin and lungs. From the experiments and experience of many physicists and physiologists, it is now ascertained that an adult would require three thousand feet of pure air, supplied every hour, in order to maintain the atmosphere of a room of an area of one thousand cubic feet in a normal state of purity.

Ventilation, which means the admission of pure air, is, therefore, a necessity to the life of all animals; and from this we can logically deduce that the length of life of people inhabiting dwellings is in proportion to the introduction therein of pure air.

The rooms that we inhabit, and particularly those that are constantly occupied by children, or by people whose vocation does not permit easy and frequent transition from one place to another, and the rooms that are not provided with sufficient ventilation, require much care from those who have the charge of them; particularly for the sake of the children, who need pure air for health and growth.

The atmosphere of inhabited rooms, when not freely ventilated, is found to contain too great a proportion of carbonic acid to be healthy; for every person inhabiting the same will give out on an average fifteen cubic feet of carbonic acid in twenty-four hours.

The normal proportion of this noxious gas contained in the air is, in volume, about one to twenty-five hundred feet, and in that diluted quantity it is innocuous; but suppose a room twenty by twenty-five, nine feet high, occupied by five persons, seventy-five cubit feet of carbonic acid would, in twenty-four hours, be given out in exchange for the oxygen of that atmosphere, and if the ventilation be not adequate to replace that oxygen and greatly dilute the carbonic acid, that atmosphere would be deadly. It must not be forgotten, too, that the air of inhabited rooms will, besides, contain scaly epithelium from the skin and from the lungs; fibres of cotton, linen or wool; particles of articles of food, wood or coal; minute hairs or parts of hairs; emanations from wall paper, particularly if damp, as mildew, fungi, and, if the paper be green, probably arsenic.

Sleeping in a close room, unless it be of very large dimensions, is unhealthy. Any one having visited a bed-room which has had the doors and windows closed during the night, and is not of very large dimensions, must have experienced the heaviness and closeness of the air, if a person has spent the night therein. It is loaded with the poison exhaled from the body of that person.

Other causes, besides the above mentioned, are conducive to the contamination of the atmosphere of rooms. Fire, gas, candles, and anything, in fact, burning, consumes oxygen and gives off carbonic acid.

The following will serve as illustrations:

Coal in combustion, gives out carbon, carbonic acid, carbonic oxide, sulphur and sulphurous compounds, as sulphuretted-hydrogen, ammonium sulphide, water, &c.

Wood, carbonic acid, oxide of carbon, and water in large quantities. It is also estimated that one pound of wood would require one hundred and twenty cubic feet of air for complete combustion.

Coal-gas, for lighting purposes, consumes from six to eight cubic feet of oxygen to the foot of gas, and produces about two cubic feet of carbonic acid and from two to five grains of sulphurous acid. Moreover, one foot of gas will consume, in burning, about eight cubic feet of air.

Gas is an article of consumption which needs all the attention possible from the consumer, for it is seldom supplied by the manufacturers in such a state of purity as to be harmless. Impure gas will emanate carbonic oxide, sulphur-compounds and proportions of ammonia, dangerous to persons exposed to them. The great injury from gas, however, is from the imperfect combustion caused by defective burners. Whenever the gas flame is blue or ragged, combustion is imperfect, and elements of gas escape. The flame should be a wide one, that the air may have free access to the particles of carbon within it. A small, round, high flame has not surface enough, and the constituents of the gas escape in an incandescent state. The habit of partially turning off the gas is a mistaken notion of economy, saving nothing, and rendering it dangerous. The illuminating power of gas is due to the quantity of oxygen allowed to have access to the particles of carbon contained in it. Therefore, a flame of a small surface allows but little oxygen to reach the particles of carbon which must escape unburnt and in a heated state.

Oil in combustion. Half an ounce of burning oil will consume over three cubic feet of the oxygen of the air, and produce half a cubic foot of carbonic acid. One pound of oil requires 160 cubic feet of air for combustion. *Candles*, and any *fat*, would, in a state of combustion, consume as much air, and produce as much carbonic acid. All the products of burning carbon are heavy, and do not rise high in the atmosphere. This is practically and largely demonstrated in manufacturing towns, as Pittsburgh, London, Manchester and others, where these products are suspended in the atmosphere in such large proportion as to blacken the houses, furniture and garments with remarkable quickness.

Under these circumstances, and, as man cannot provide for the cooking of his food, an agreeable warm temperature in winter and light at night, without the use of articles of combustion, ventilation becomes imperative. The air of dwellings must be constantly renewed, and that can only be done through doors and windows, or such ventilators as skillful mechanics have invented for the purpose. Spacious rooms, with high ceilings, preserve the purity of the atmosphere, inasmuch as the exhalations of the body, and the products of combustion, would take longer to taint it with impurities, than they would to taint that of rooms of a smaller area.

Another source of impurity of air in dwellings, and particularly in the expensive ones of the richer class, is the *water-closet*, the *bath-tub*, the *stationary basin* connected with the sewer. The sewer-traps, intended to prevent the rising of sewer gases into the rooms, do not accomplish that object, particularly in cities exposed to high and low tides; for, during high tide the river water will enter the mouth of the sewers, preventing not only the escape of the gases, but actually forcing them backwards and upwards. The amount of water in the traps is not sufficient to resist the pressure, and the gases bubble up through it, and enter the rooms through the apertures of the water-closet, bath-tubs and stationary wash-basins. To cure this defect permanently a flue should be connected with the sewer before it enters the house. The flue, like a water spout, might be made of tin, and attached to a wall of the house, or even made to enter a chimney flue; but it should rise above the roof, and fully as high as the chimney-tops. All returning sewer-gases will then find an easy exit through this ventilator, and the small amount of gas remaining between the place connecting the sewer with the ventilator, and the trap just below the water-closet or basin would be prevented from entering the room by the water in the trap.

The air of rooms occupied by the sick is generally vitiated by the abundant exhalations from their bodies, and by emanations from the discharged secretions. Pathologists now declare that the rapid infection of cholera and yellow fever has its source in the emanations of the fecal matter of the patient; ozone, the great oxidizing agent of the air, is scarcely ever found in the atmosphere of sick rooms. The plausible reason is that the impurities require so much ozone for their oxidation that none is left free. Whether this is true or not the fact remains that ozone is never found in foul atmospheres, or in atmospheres tainted by the exhalations of swampy grounds; while it is found in abundance in pure air, particularly of the mountains and of the sea.

The sick room, then, should be kept well ventilated at all times; but particularly so when occupied by persons affected with skin diseases, as scarlet fever, measles, chicken pox, varioloid, small pox, erysipelas; or by zymotic diseases, as typhoid fever; or by cholera, pulmonary consumption, diphtheria, etc.

It has already been stated that the normal quantity of carbonic acid in the air is, as to volume, one to twenty-five hundred cubic feet of air. Roscoe, however, found that the air of a school-room occupied by 67 boys, (69 cubic feet of space per head), contained more than three parts of carbonic acid to 1,000. Weaver, in examining a room occupied by six persons, (51 cubic feet of space per head), with three jets of gas burning, found more than five parts of carbonic acid to 1,000 feet of air; and Pettenkofer found that the air of a school-room occupied by 70 girls, (150 cubic feet of space per head), contained the enormous quantity of seven parts of carbonic acid to 1,000 cubic feet of air.

The disparity in the proportions above given being mainly due to the greater or less quantity of air allowed to enter into those rooms, it is readily seen that even the least vitiated of those atmospheres would be harmful to the persons breathing them; for it should not be forgotten that besides the carbonic acid other impurities must exist, as before mentioned.

Considering all the circumstances of impurities of the air, and the fact that girls remain longer and oftener within rooms than boys, it is reasonable to deduce the inference that the ventilation of houses is of peculiar importance to that them.

Girls at school, and particularly at the age of puberty, when their organism is eminently sensitive, suffer greatly from confined air. It is, therefore, incumbent upon parents to visit the school-rooms often, and see that proper and adequate ventilation is secured.

The bedrooms of girls need also particular attention, for girls are apt to spend much of their time in them. Let such rooms be not only freely ventilated, but exposed to the sun if possible.

It is well known that persons breathing air rendered

impure by respiration, by the exhalations of the body, and evaporations of the skin, leading a sedentary life, or remaining in a constrained position several hours at a time become anæmic; lose their appetite, are subject to headache, and loss of strength. This is the first step towards pulmonary consumption. Girls at puberty require pure air; a perfect oxygenation of their blood is conducive to the naturalness of all their functions, and particularly of menstruation.

In the following few words of Angus Smith we find food enough for reflection on this subject: "It must be remembered that the parts of which we are composed are continually undergoing change; the blood and the fluids are especially active. Let us picture to ourselves the amount of this activity. If we hold our breath a few seconds we are uncomfortable, a little more and we are unconscious; if we inhale a little undiluted sulphuretted hydrogen we fall down unconscious, as if struck by lightning; if we inhale even carbonic oxide, which we cannot smell, we fall down at once; by carbonic oxide obtained by combustion from an iron furnace, men have been suddenly thrown down without warning."

We would recommend that the several hints given in this article be carefully read and remembered. It is to be regretted that a volume like this could not permit a greater diffusion on this subject, for it is a very vital one. We leave it as it is, trusting that it may be sufficient to awaken amongst the intelligent that desire for a thorough knowledge that may lead them to the study of works prepared especially for a more comprehensive understanding of the subject.

PART III.

FUNCTIONAL IRREGULARITIES

AND THEIR PREVENTIVE TREATMENT.

From the moment a woman attains the age of puberty she becomes an object of solicitude to the physician. We shall consider her at that particular age of youth and beauty when the diseases that threaten her are those which greatly influence her health and happiness ever after.

CHAPTER I.

SYMPTOMS OF DISTURBANCE.

THE functions of the generative organs of woman are not always established without subjecting her to annoyances, nay, even to afflictions and sufferings, which need salutary counsel.

Woman is subject to the process of menstruation for the best period of her life. During this long term, of thirty years of her womanhood, her health is dependent on the accomplishment of that function; according to the success or failure of that process she either flourishes in the enjoyment of health or languishes in pain and weakness. A girl is seldom the subject of special anxiety until she enters the state of puberty; like a boy, she runs and plays, and nature undertakes no peculiar mode of growth suggestive of sexual individuality. Puberty, although apparently sudden, is effected gradually, and not always without accident. Its manifestation in menstruation may be so abnormal as to constitute a real malady. The mode by which this natural process is effected has been treated elsewhere. (See chapter on Puberty.)

A girl in a perfect state of health may be taken by such acute and severe symptoms as to lead one to suspect indications of a dangerous malady.

Parents, also, have been misled by the peculiar complaints into the belief that sickness was simulated, when, in reality, their daughter should have been rather an object of sympathy. Again, ignorant attendants, believing such an indisposition to be but an accidental attack of colic from indigestion or otherwise, have filled girls to drunkenness with alcoholic stimulants.

Menstrual colic having been mistaken also for a symptom of worms, or for some other imaginary ailment, medicaments, unfit for the girl's condition, have been administered, to the detriment of her general health.

It cannot be denied, however, that the symptoms are often obscure and confusing, because acute pain in the abdomen, accompanied by tightness and oppression, may suggest flatulency; irregular and heavy pain may suggest the presence of worms; yet, the age of the girl, the suddenness of the attack in the midst of good health, the periodical return of these indispositions, the regularity of the pulse, the natural condition of the skin, the cleanness of the tongue, the absence of indigestion or of diarrhœa, and the shortness of the pain should rather suggest a natural preparation for the menstrual flux. Moreover, menstrual colics are almost always attended by *coldness of the feet*.

These colics are generally relieved by hot foot-baths, application of heat over the region of the uterus: a bag of hot hops, or a hot corn-meal poultice. If there are complications, as tendency of blood to the head, neuralgias, pain in the chest, etc., some medical treatment may be required about which a physician should be consulted.

The establishment of menstruation is not unfrequently attended by serious constitutional difficulties, as chlorosis (green-sickness) and hysteria. Its manifestation may also be attended by such modifications of the general system as will result in an aggravation, or a decided amelioration, of the girl's usual condition. All of the special maladies incidental to menstruation will be treated hereafter, separately.

The appearance of the menses should be the signal for a girl to seek rest in a horizontal position, and for the avoidance of extreme cold and heat. Her beverages should be warm rather than iced. We have known a glass of ice water, taken while the body was heated by exercise, to suppress the menses instantly, and induce severe colic pains. The dress should be easy, loose around the chest and abdomen. Linen-wear should be discarded at such times, for it is too great a conductor of heat, allowing the body to cool too rapidly.

Delicate and nervous persons should adopt a system calculated to improve the general health; as exercise in the open air, riding on horseback, taking trips to the country. If inclined to melancholy they should seek distraction in innocent pleasures, and in the company of congenial friends.

During the period of menstruation woman should be an object of solicitude, for even her moral nature may, during that time, be exposed to changes which appear extraordinary to an observer. One author says that it is seldom that menstruation occurs without inducing some change in the usual demeanor of women. The majority of them are subject to weariness, vague desires, melancholy; they may be more irritable in their manners, more impressionable, easily frightened and discouraged; they are also more liable to take cold and more susceptible to the changes of the weather; in other words, they are the victims of many little infirmities, which ought to be recognized and treated with kindness, rather than ridicule. Those who are naturally sensitive should be surrounded by soothing influences, and not exposed to anything that exalts the imagination. The diet should be light, and free from rich condiments and stimulating spices. The bath should be warm, and under no circumstances should the body be immersed in cold water immediately before the appearance of menstruation or during its continuance, even though it had been the habit to do so at other times. The feet should always be kept warm and dry.

Women of lymphatic temperament, of scanty menstruation, should be nourished generously with rare beef, roasted or broiled; rich soups, particularly of peas and beans. A little light wine, as claret or sherry, would be beneficial. Such women should also dress warmly, occupying well ventilated apartments, and make repeated excursions to the country.

Mothers should be particularly attentive to instruct their girls at the time when the generative functions are likely to commence; for it has often occurred that the unexpected appearance of blood on the garments has frightened girls into serious illnesses. It is also necessary that they should be made acquainted with all the causes that may produce suppression or derangement. Ignorance has often led girls into errors which they would have avoided, had they known the serious consequences that would follow. Exposure to the inclemency of the weather, dampness, heat or cold; excessive exercise in walking, dancing, riding, playing or otherwise; exposing the heated body to a draught of cold air;

plunging the feet into cold water; a sudden emotion, as fright, passion, joy; a violent pain; a drink of ice-water, particularly when the body is warm; a sudden check of perspiration—may induce immediate suppression and all its concomitant painful results.

In recapitulating the indispositions to which a young girl may be exposed during the period of menstruation, an author says: "If she is strong and robust, she may be tormented with vertigo, motes before her eyes, buzzing in her ears, flashes of heat in her face, nervous or congestive headache, sleeplessness, and even convulsions. Her eyes may be congested, and shed tears easily; her pulse bouncing and frequent; her temporal arteries throb; she may be subject to palpitation of the heart; to bleeding of the nose; to impeded respiration, and to sighing. She may be generally oppressed, or subject to pains and colic, and to fatigue from the least exercise. If she is feeble and lymphatic, she may be subject to congestion of the head, although her face may be pale, her eyes languid, her pulse weak and slow;—also to palpitation of the heart, but not so violent as in the sanguine temperament. Her digestion may be feeble, yet she may desire indigestible substances, and sometimes articles entirely unfit for her condition. She may be subject to heaviness in the region of the stomach, to lassitude, to weakness even, and to the flow of leucorrhœa." So that the occurrence of symptoms like these, at the time of life spoken of, need not be looked on as alarming, but should, nevertheless, be carefully watched and attended to.

We have no intention of making this a medical treatise which may impart an intimate knowledge of causes and effects, and of preventive and curative means of treating *all* diseases peculiar to women; but a general review of some of these topics will be given which we trust will be of assistance in the preservation of health, and especially that of young girls, who are yet in time for precaution and proper care in advance. And in this, the reader will not be impatient at some repetitions or renewed applications of facts and ideas already treated of. "Line upon line" is the teacher's surest road to the intelligent understanding of the learners.

CHAPTER II.

CAUSES OF FUNCTIONAL DERANGEMENT.

THESE causes may be divided into two classes:— *Remote* and *Immediate*. Under the first head let us consider several points.

1. *Temperaments* (see chapter on "Temperaments,") are often the predisposing cause of diseases of the menstrual organs. Women of lymphatic and nervous-lymphatic temperament are more prone to scanty menstruation, to leucorrhœa ("whites"), and hysteria, while the sanguine or nervous-sanguine temperaments are more liable to excessive and to painful menstruation. Where the nervous temperament predominates, the susceptibility to excitement and to external impression predisposes the individual to conditions which disturb the natural exercise of the menstrual functions. The hygiene of temperaments has already been treated under their respective chapters.

2. *Diet and nourishment.* In the article on food this subject has been fully discussed. But we may add here that *insufficient, excessive,* or *improper food*, disturbing the equilibrium of the vital forces, deranging the stomach, affecting the heart and the circulation, may induce such irritability of the nervous system as to predispose the organs of generation to functional derangements.

Insufficiency of nourishment impoverishes the blood, lessens the vital force, weakens the action of the heart in the distribution of blood; and in the general insufficiency of the circulation of that all-important fluid the ovaries and the womb become the participants, manifesting their disorder in the scanty, pale, watery menstrual fluids, in leucorrhœa, and the relaxation of the muscles of the womb and its ligaments.

Excess of food, on the other hand, overtasks the functions of the stomach, distends its capacity as well as that of the intestines, and finally weakens digestion and the power of assimilation. Blood increases in quantity, distending the vessels and inducing general plethora. Excess of food then, and, particularly, if composed of highly seasoned dishes, overloads and irritates the system, until the womb and the ovaries, overcome by the plethora and irritability incidental to that condition, express their abnormal condition by painful menstruation, irritable uterus, etc.

On the subject of inordinate indulgence, we prefer allowing a lady to speak for herself. As far back as sixty years ago she wrote to a young friend: "A young beauty, were she as fair as Hebe, and elegant as the Goddess of Love herself, would soon lose these charms by a course of immoderate eating, drinking, and late hours. Some of my readers may start at the idea, and wonder how it can be, that any lady could be guilty of either immoderate eating or drinking. But when I speak of inordinate eating, etc., I do not mean feasting like a glutton, or drinking to intoxication. My objection is not more against the quantity than the quality of the dishes which constitute the usual repast of women of fashion. Their breakfast not only sets forth tea, coffee, and chocolate, but hot bread and butter. The last two, when taken constantly, are hostile to health and female delicacy. The heated grease which is their principal ingredient deranges the stomach. After this meal, a long and exhausting fast not unfrequently succeeds, from nine or ten in the morning until six or seven o'clock in the evening, when dinner is served up; and the half famished beauty sits down to sate a keen appetite with spiced soups, fish, roast and boiled meats, game, tarts, sweetmeats, ices, fruits, &c. How must the constitution suffer under the digestion of this *mélange!* How does the heated complexion bear witness to the combustion within!

"The superabundance of aliment which she takes in at this time is not only destructive to beauty, but the period of such repletion is full of other dangers. Long fasting wastes the powers of digestion and weakens the spring of life. In this enfeebled state, at the hour when nature intends you should prepare for general repose, you put your stomach and animal spirits to extraordinary exertion; your vital forces are overtasked and overloaded, and thus every complaint that distresses and destroys the human frame may be engendered. I am fully persuaded that long fasting, late dinners, and the repletion then taken into the stomach, with the tight pressure of stiffened stays on the most susceptible part of the frame then called into action, and the midnight, nay, morning hours of lingering pleasure, are positive causes of disease; and delicate proportions give place either to miserable leanness or shapeless fat; the once fair skin assumes a pallid rigidity, or a bloated redness which the vain possessor would still regard as the roses of health. To repair these ravages, comes the aid of padding to give shape where there is none, stays to compress into form the chaos of flesh, and paints of all hues to rectify the disorder of the complexion. But useless are these attempts."

We cannot but indorse this logical lady; we grant her the privilege of speaking authoritatively; to her recital may be added more specifically that the unrestrained indulgence, so graphically set forth by her, excites the nervous and sexual system and engenders especially maladies of the menstrual organs, which are distressing and debilitating in the extreme. Every inordinate stimulation is inevitably followed by reaction, which is weakness and disability.

3. *Vitiated air* is another source of the general debility of women, and of derangements of their menstrual functions. The reader will find this subject treated at length in chapters on "Air," and "Hygiene to preserve the health of women."

4. *Want of exercise and indolence* stand foremost among the causes of uterine and ovarian derangements. Exercise is the harmonizer between the supply and the consumption, in other words, between nourishment and wear-and-tear. When properly conducted it gives vigor and strength to the body and assists all the organs in the performance of their functions. Deprive woman of sun, air, and exercise, and she becomes enervated; the functions of her generative organs languish; she loses her bright tints and colors, general debility follows, and in the general breaking down the menstrual organs assume maladies that add to the irritation and discomfort of the girl.

"If a young woman," a physician says, "would be well-shaped and well-conditioned, and would escape

FUNCTIONAL DERANGEMENT.

pains and the doctor, if she would have grace and elasticity of movement, color in her cheeks, and admirable proportions in her limbs; if she would have a faultless foot and ankle, limbs of swelling proportion, the flesh firm, and the shape such as no sculptor could improve"—to which we add: if she would escape the thousand and one annoyances, pains and indispositions of deranged menstruation, or of irritable womb and ovaries—"she must avail herself of sunshine and use due exercise *on foot*. Three, four, five, or six miles a day is not any too much for a woman in respectable health. Horseback riding is an excellent auxiliary, but carriage riding is *too lazy* an exercise to do much good."

The various modes of exercise and their relation to health will be found in the chapter on "Exercise" (p. 114).

5. *Mind and Imagination.* The reflex action of the operations of the mind on the generative organs is so direct and immediate that over-exertion of the intellect and the prurient habits of the imagination rank preeminent among the predisposing causes of uterine and ovarian diseases. The ambition of parents to have a girl excel in mental development at an age when nature demands her freedom for physical growth, and the establishment of the functions special to her sex, has sacrificed many a lovely maiden to an untimely grave.

Physiologists and humanitarians have devoted much time and study to the education of woman, and particularly in relation to the functional disorders of her sex. To Dr. Edward M. Clark thanks should be tendered for his admirable essays on "Sex in Education" and "The Building of a Brain." His investigations are thorough, his arguments are unanswerable. We recommend all parents to carefully peruse those priceless volumes. Unwilling to rely upon his own observations alone, he has consulted eminent medical authorities, superintendents of schools and teachers, and it is wonderful to notice the unanimity of opinion on this subject among persons unknown to each other, and in different pursuits of life. The State Board of Health of Massachusetts has also added its valuable quota to the important information.

From all these sources we learn that girls at school, submissive to strict discipline, restricted in bodily exercise by reason (social) of their sex, rendered emulous by competition with boys in the higher studies of science or mathematics, become victims of overstrained mental powers, of over-excited nervous systems, and perish from the withdrawal of too much nervous force. Languor and exhaustion overcome them, the functions of the viscera and of the menstrual organs especially are impaired, and a life of strength and health is changed to one of pain and misery.

Among the many and illustrious correspondents of Dr. Clark, one says: "This baleful result becomes very strikingly manifested as the girls approach the age of puberty. Under the abnormal conditions of the physical system produced by this cause, not only do the more emulous and studious girls suffer from the study which they evidently ought to intermit; but the ordinary and habitual task-work necessary to keep abreast of the studies is far too severe a draught on many constitutions."

Another says: "Girls suffer more than boys from attendance at school. Were, however, the habits of the two sexes the same in regard to out-door play and exercise, there would probably be no difference between the power of resistance in one and the other sex till the approach of puberty. As a girl draws near this period, menstruates, and becomes capable of child-bearing, the school discipline and work must bend to her bodily needs in a manner not required by boys. Her menstrual week must be respected. During these days her mental powers are easily overstrained. The depressing influence of confinement in the school-room, long continued standing, or even sitting, do her bodily harm."

Professor Elias Loomis, of Yale College, in his report in which he speaks so highly of the mental qualities of woman, of her wonderful achievements even in the world of science, represents that her physical nature suffers under the great strain of emulation, and closes in this wise: " As we look upon the increasing physical deterioration of our American girls, and reflect that they are to become the mothers of an unborn generation, on which will surely fall an inheritance of defective physical organization and consequent mental infirmities, it is time to sound a note of alarm, and look at the causes which are undermining the Republic, and search for the remedies that should be applied. . . In conclusion let me say, that we are a people given to experiment. There is nothing in our politics, economies, or religion that must not be put to the "*experimentum crucis.*" This is true of our schools for girls. . . . The cry to our older colleges and time-honored universities is, Open your doors, that the fairer part of creation may enter and join in the mental tilt and tournament. God save the American people from such a misfortune!"

Dr. William A. Hammond says: "Puberty being a

much more complex process in girls than in boys, the former are more liable to disease at this time; and this liability is increased by whatever tends still more to exhaust the nervous system, such as mental application and anxiety. I have repeatedly seen cases in which the flow of the menses had been suddenly stopped by the anxiety induced by the necessity of learning a school lesson."

While we could cite many authorities to prove the baneful effects of excessive mental labor in girls, we will close by reproducing, from Dr. Clark's work on *The Building of a Brain*, a mother's letter upon the sad fate of her daughter. The plain and graphic story is simple and full of instruction, and warmed as it is by the pathetic throbs of a mother's heart, it conveys an irresistible truth that should be heard by every parent:

"At the age of fifteen Mary was a remarkably fine and healthy girl; she seemed to be safely over the critical period, and, until after that time, had never suffered as many girls do at the commencement of their womanhood. Her thinking powers were quick and vigorous; and she was the pride of her teachers and the joy of her parents. Unlimited mental progress was laid out before her, and it seemed that there were to be no bounds to her acquirements.

"She had then finished a good common school education, at the best high school, and had entered an institute for young ladies, of the highest character. The curriculum of study there was comprehensive, and it required the closest application of an ambitious scholar to succeed.

"One hour was allowed for walking and recreation

during the day; and half of that could be spent, if the pupil desired to do so, in the music room. As the months went on, I began to notice that her complexion, which had been pure rose leaf, became almost transparent, and that the fresh blood left her cheeks; still she did not complain, nor lose flesh, but said sometimes, that if she could *sleep a week*, she would enjoy it, and that it almost always happened when she was unwell she had the most to do, and the longest to stand. Her progress in her studies was wonderful; and it seems incredible to me now that we should have allowed her to devote herself to them so entirely. Her musical talents were great, and they were under cultivation also; when she was seventeen she was the first soprano singer in the choir of the church to which she belonged.

"At last I began to be alarmed at the remarkable flow whenever she was unwell, and at the *frequent recurrence of the periodical function.* [The italics are ours.] I felt as if something should be done, and consulted our family physician as to what could be given her, and how this increased action could be stopped or diminished. He prescribed iron as a tonic, but said that we should do nothing more; for that 'every woman was a law unto herself,' and as long as nothing more serious occurred, she was to be let alone. This from a man who had daughters himself, and eminent in the profession! Never a word about rest, never a caution that she could overwork herself, and thus bring misery for the remainder of her life. She left school, in June of that year, with noble honors and aching frame; and after two months' vacation and rest, which seemed to do her a world of good, began in September another year of unremitting, hard study. Loving and gratified parents, proud and expectant teachers, looked upon her as capable of accomplishing all that had ever been done by faithful students, and of advancing far beyond all who were in the graduating class with her. Her teachers were as kind as any could have been. I think the fault was in the system that requires so many hours of study, no matter what the condition of the pupil may be.

"As an instance: twenty-five questions were given her to be answered. She was seated at a table, without books, from 10 A. M. till 3 P. M., ceaselessly *thinking* and writing; and the twenty-five questions in classical literature were faultlessly answered, and that, too, at a time when, had I known what I now know, she should have been resting on her bed. Her father, to whom the paper was shown for approval, wrote on the margin: 'It seems to me that the task imposed here was a *great one indeed;* but it has been performed with good success.'

"I do not for a moment mean to find fault with her teachers; for kinder, more interested ones no pupil ever had; and the delight that a teacher derives from a painstaking and appreciative pupil cannot be understood by those unused to teaching.

"While the dear child was meeting our utmost requirements as a scholar, the foundation of her life was being sapped away.

"In May, 1872, a little more than two weeks before the June commencement, she was taken with fearful sickness and severe chills, just after one of the hemorrhages which came every three weeks regularly. [Menstrual, of course.] Our doctor was called; the first thing she said to him was, 'Doctor, I must not be sick now. I cannot afford the time. I must be well for commencement.' For four days she suffered very much, but quinine and all sorts of tonics brought her up; and the two weeks that should have been taken to get well in were spent in study, study, study. All the examinations were passed successfully, even brilliantly; and she was graduated with all the honors of the institution. Oh, how proud we were of her! and when she came home, frail and weak as a wilted flower, we said that she should have a long rest, and every comfort that we could give her. All summer she remained in the highlands of the Hudson; yet, when autumn came, she was not as well as we thought she ought to be, though very much improved with regard to *the monthly turns, they recurring at right times now*.

"In September she commenced studying again; her French and music were continued, so that she might become still more accomplished in those branches; and lectures on rhetoric and moral philosophy were attended also.

"The habit of studying was so strong upon her that she could not give it up. Now came swelling of the joints and fingers, and the *old trouble*, all of which she would have kept to herself if she could have done so; but I was so anxious about her that I ascertained her condition, went to the doctor again, and begged him to tell me what to do that would stop the weakening *periodical disturbance*, as I was persuaded that was the cause of her trouble. He said she had inflammatory rheumatism, and prescribed *soda*. But I was not to do anything for the other matter, and, against my own convictions, I let things take their course. Oh, if he had said, 'Take her home, and stop her studying.' Armed with such authority, I would have done it; and how do we know but she might have been with us now, if I had done so? But she worked on until the 25th of December. Then she came home, and said decidedly she would study no more till she was *well*.

"We were rejoiced at her decision; for although we were anxious that her education should be complete and thorough, we had felt for a long time that her health was becoming impaired. Still we were sure she had a good constitution, and that would carry her through. She did not grow thin, but *stout* and pale; and such a transparent pallor that, now I think of it, I wonder all who looked at her did not see that her blood was turning to water. Her sweet and lovely soul was so uncomplaining, and her smile always so bright, that we never for a moment thought she could *fade* and *die*.

"She brightened up somewhat for the next month, but still did not get well. About the last of January her limbs swelled so much that, in haste, I rushed to the doctor. Then he said her kidneys were congested, and that Bright's fatal disease was her malady. All that despairing love could do was done *now*. In five short weeks we laid her in Greenwood. Whatever was the form of disease from which she suffered, I am convinced that what she did have was brought on by excessive study, *when she should have rested*, and that it was fixed at the time when she got the severe chills, May, 1871.

"She was by no means a frail girl when she entered the institute. She was tall, finely formed, with a full, broad chest, and musical organs of great compass. Her bust was not flat, neither was it as full as might have been. Her features were not too large. She had brown eyes, brown hair, a very sweet and pleasing face. With every indication at first of strength and good constitution, she fell at last a victim to want of sense in parents, and teachers, and (shall I say?) physicians, too."

We make no apology for transferring here this letter in full. Besides sympathizing with this broken-hearted woman, which would be sufficient reason for us to send abroad every word of her lament, we feel that a more comprehensive, true, and significant illustration of the carelessness in educating girls could not be given by the most experienced and observant hygienist.

Body and mind being parts of a grand whole, reflecting and depending upon each other, to neglect one is to injure the other simultaneously; exceptions form no valid argument against the requirements of this general law. Infringe it, and the penalty sooner or later must be paid. A proper equilibrium should be maintained by exercising the body and the mind, alternately with periods of rest and nourishment, necessary to the recovery of vitality lost in the exercise of mental or physical attributes.

6. *Exposure to wet, heat, or cold.* These predisposing causes to functional derangements of the female organs are set forth in the chapters on "Clothing" and "Air." Getting wet at the times when the periods are about to appear, or are actually on, is probably more of an immediate than a remote cause of menstrual derangement. It will be treated under the paragraph on "Immediate causes."

7. *Impedimenta.* All kinds of mechanical pressure, as in the appliance of tight clothing, is another predispos-

ing cause, affecting the circulation and the natural development of the muscular system. (See "Clothing.")

8. *Uncleanliness.* "Cleanliness is next to godliness." What a remarkable adage! Why is cleanliness considered so excellent as to be reckoned next to virtue? Is it because uncleanliness is repulsive to the human sense? That would be the negative reason The proposition is, that cleanliness, mental, as well as physical, is purity—purity of the mind, purity of the body. Impurities of the skin engender disease. The skin is an organ of absorption and secretion: it absorbs from the surrounding atmosphere elements of vitality; it secretes effete fluids of the body. It is the safety-valve during excesses of temperature; it contracts when exposed to a very cold atmosphere, preventing the blood of the capillaries from becoming suddenly chilled, and secretes fluid when exposed to a high temperature, inducing evaporation and cooling, thus preventing congestion. Uncleanliness of this organ is a mechanical obstruction to its natural function, the bad effect of which reflects upon the whole system. It should be kept clean and protected from the excesses of temperature. When chilled suddenly it has caused dangerous congestions, checked or stopped the flow of the menses; and when it is kept for a long time in an unclean state, or exposed to sudden heat or cold, it becomes a source of chronic ailments of the chest and of the menstrual organs. (See "Air," "Clothing," and "Circulation.")

8. *Occupation* is always a source of health, while its negative, *Idleness*, is generally a source of disease. Among the class in which the mental faculties are excited to premature activity, and the body is allowed to

remain inactive, an unwonted irritability of the nervous system is the consequence. The harmonious, self-possessed cheerfulness of the woman of physical labor compares favorably with the faulty temper, fretfulness and weariness of the girl of indolence. The sleeplessness, headache, nausea, loss of appetite, abdominal pains, backache, and general good-for-nothingness of the latter, is seldom found in the former. The life of the idler is emotional; the life of the worker is practical. The ailings of the nervous, indolent girl are soothed only by romantic literature, which excites the senses that reflect upon her organs of generation; the active girl overcomes the senses by a healthy exercise of the physical, and finds vigor in peaceful rest.

The occupations calculated to injure girls are such as demand an unwonted strain upon the abdominal muscles, *e. g.*, standing too long—as shop girls at a counter—long practice at the sewing-machine, or sitting too long bent over a desk. Girls at school, keeping a sitting posture for six hours, wearing stays, which, on account of their stiffness, must press the abdomen inwardly whenever the body is bent forward upon itself, are liable to displacements of the womb from undue pressure. And even if the womb is not displaced the circulation of the abdomen is interfered with, which is then manifested in the costiveness of the intestines, and in painful menstruation from irritability of the ovaries.

IMMEDIATE CAUSES.

When any of the foregoing Remote or *predisposing* causes exist, menstrual derangement is easily brought about, even by a slight exciting cause or immediate occasion.

1. *Exposure* to a sudden change from heat to cold, getting the feet or the body wet while dressed, allowing the wet clothes to evaporate and dry while on the person, will abstract so much heat from the body as to cause a shock to the system that may induce immediate suppression of the menses with all its evil consequences. And when this is repeated, inflammation of the ovaries and uterus will follow, capable of putting life in immediate peril, or of exposing to such derangements of the menstrual organs as will consign a girl to months and years of suffering.

2. *Emotions*. A sudden mental excitement from joy, sorrow, or fright often as suddenly checks the flow, producing a dangerous retention. "The menstrual organs are especially susceptible to the influence of excitement of the passions, and their disorders are *oftener traceable to this source than to any other.*" The pleasures of society, inebriating to the young girl; her entrance to the theatre of love and passion, the fascination of erotic literature, dramas, or scenes, are often the beginning of a series of evils that sap her mind and destroy her body. Woman, by nature, more emotional than man, aggravating her condition by the effort to conceal what she fears may endanger her dignity, is rendered more susceptible to the evil consequences that result from the excitability of the senses.

The mother has evidently a serious duty to perform here. She should watch her daughter's associates; shield her from luxury and fashion; withdraw from her all literature of doubtful morality; restrain her from all things that fever the imagination, from intemperate wishes, from the enchantment of the senses. Unremitting vigilance, confidence and love should be her weapons. Purity of thought, tranquillity of heart and mind, will save her daughter from the gulf of errors to which she unconsciously tends, and where she will find only misery for her soul and destruction for her body.

At a certain period of life, the purest heart and the mind most chaste are susceptible to the passion of love. With melancholic, dreamy, indolent natures, it is a fiery ordeal. Civilization has elevated the passion of the savage into a sentiment of affection in the refined. An ardent love, even in the latter, can take possession of the soul, agitate and dominate it. The younger and purer the heart, the stronger the affection which may be kindled into a passion by the enervating atmosphere of ball-rooms, theaters, toilets and perfumes that fascinate the senses. Socrates said: "The wind nourishes the fire; habit and opportunity inflame love." An inordinate love, engaging wholly the imagination, is fraught with danger to the celibate; it engenders disorders that affect the entire human economy; the surexcitation of the senses induces feverishness, restlessness, anxiety, sleeplessness, loss of appetite, melancholy; and nervous persons, tender and innocent girls, building a world of their own imagination, rising above the vulgar earth into a sentimental sphere, where daily avocations and animal necessities are too coarse to be observed, waste in flesh and droop in spirit, until maladies of a serious nature overtake them: hysteria, melancholy, chlorosis, neuralgias, etc. The organs of menstruation, in sympathy with the general abnormal condition of the system, suffer; and irritation, inflammation of the womb, leucorrhœa, may easily be the results.

Unrequited love, or strenuous opposition, is even more dangerous. It is an unequal fight; it is a struggle of the imagination against fate; it is a hopeless one. The young girl lives in the secret chamber of her fanciful architecture alone; she is sad and dreary. The roses soon leave her cheeks, she becomes pale and hollow-eyed, morbidly sensitive; sighs come deep from her very heart, and tears flow easily; general weakness finally confines her to her couch; nothing can distract her mind now; nothing attracts her from solitude; she is alone among a thousand people; the roundness of her limbs deserts her; an irritating cough makes its appearance, fever (hectic) follows, and the grave in the dim distance opens its doors for her to enter.

Parents often fail in the manner of training girls whose attachments they disapprove. Fathers are too often harsh, and mothers whine over an imaginary ingratitude of the girl; how could she love anyone but her father and mother who have reared her, been so indulgent to her? etc. It is wonderful how a full stomach forgets the keen sensation of hunger! Although the girl is already, by the very affection of which they complain, disabled from thinking and judging rightly of the fitness of things, or of considering coolly and philosophically while passion is burning, she is expected to act with reason and circumspection. Father and mother might better look back and see in the mirror of their own life the very reflection of the daughter's condition. Sternness and bitter reproaches are out of place now, and certainly unavailing, as has been proved a thousand times. Travelling, change of scene, sympathy, love and good companionship, will do more towards calming the troubled spirit, and cooling the feverish excitement, than all the arguments or modes of coercion possible.

The all-powerful guard against dangerous emotions, or reveries, is *habitual occupation*. *Habitual* is written understandingly, for transient occupation is not calculated to engage the mind; but, when habitual, it becomes a necessity, on account of which it is performed, even though the mind is preoccupied by thoughts foreign to the act. It is this habitual occupation that so often enables man to withstand emotions that disappointments and misfortunes induce; the dignity of labor, the interest in his profession or trade, the healthful effort to succeed, and pride in conquering adversity, make him powerful in the struggle for existence. If a woman is so devoted to the duties of her vocation as to render her life a necessity to others, or, to such pursuits as engage her intellect in the accomplishment of something worthy of herself and of the respect of her fellow-creatures, in either case, allegiance to her higher nature is evinced by self-forgetfulness and loving care for others in the one, and manifestations of a healthy active brain in the other, and she is not the victim of passion or sentimentality.

Let every girl have an *habitual* occupation with which she is identified for success or failure, and the problem of life will become to her a fact of practical value, instead of a sentimental illusion. Let her be one of the helping hands of the household; let her be identified with all the interests and struggles of her parents; let her employment be steady and progressive, and she will not seek rest or solace from her "ennui" in the romances of the day, in the admiration of silly youths, nor in the vanity of ever-changing fashion. Conscious of her usefulness, she will respect herself, which is to have the strongest bulwark against the insidious attacks of imaginary evils, or excessive and unhappy emotions.

ACCIDENTAL AND OTHER CAUSES.

An injury, a fall, a shot, a railroad accident not in any way fatal, will cause a shock to the nervous system that may induce a sudden suppression of the menses. Acute diseases, as fever, hemorrhoidal hemorrhage, inflammation of the bowels, dysentery, pneumonia, pleurisy, etc., often induce a suppression, not only during the acuteness of the disease, but even until the general system has totally recovered from the debilitating influence. Change of climate, particularly from a high to a low temperature, and brought about in a quick manner; travelling—crossing high mountains, and even crossing the sea—has induced suppression of menstruation. There is no doubt that the cause is found in the quick succession of change in the temperature or other conditions of the atmosphere. It has also happened that women who lived in level districts and menstruated regularly were subject to suppression of menses while residing on high mountains, or at sea; and that the return did not occur even for several months after change of locality. Novelty of situation, change of exercise, as, going to live in a house having many steps to ascend and descend, or even so slight a thing as changing from carpeted steps to marble ones, has sometimes caused temporary suspensions.

The natural suspension of menstruation, the critical period that occurs at a certain time of life (at about the age of forty-five), is the cessation of reproduction, commonly called "change of life." It is a natural process and should be unattended by discomfort or illness, but alas! the hygienic rules so long disobeyed bring their result even at this stage, consequently, the process of cessation is hardly ever undergone without entailing upon woman disease and suffering.

Another natural suppression is pregnancy. (See author's *Maternity*.)

CHAPTER III.

AMENORRHŒA.

DELAYED MENSTRUATION. SUPPRESSION, AND RETENTION OF THE MENSES. CHLOROSIS.

AMENORRHŒA means *absence of the menses*, and is therefore used as the generic term for the three disorders, *suppressed*, *retained*, and *delayed* menstruation, although each is distinct from the others, having causes and effects peculiar to itself. Many of the symptoms of these disorders are alike, but a close and comparative examination will show the distinctive features of each, the knowledge of which is important to a proper discrimination in the selection of the means to avert them.

DELAYED MENSTRUATION.

By the above term might be understood a tardy ap-appearance of the usual flow; but in this connection it is used to mean the *non-appearance of the menses at the time of life when it is reasonable to suppose they should be manifested*. In the chapter on "Puberty," it has already been stated that in warm latitudes this climacteric change would occur from the tenth to the fourteenth year, in temperate ones from the twelfth to the sixteenth, and in northern regions from the fourteenth to the eighteenth. When these periods in the life of girls pass away, taking into consideration the respective latitudes, and this process of puberty is not manifested, menstruation has been unreasonably *delayed*, and becomes, therefore, a subject of great interest and solicitude.

Menstruation may be impossible, as in the case of congenital malformation in which the ovaries, the womb, or the vagina, are absent; or, in cases of disorganization from violent inflammations in which adhesions of the walls of the vagina, or of the mouth of the womb, have taken place; in the case of imperforation of the hymen. These cases are rare, but they do sometimes occur.

The causes more common for this delay are, however, constitutional rather than organic, and generally yield to hygienic and medical treatment. There are instances in which a tendency to a late establishment of this function is hereditary, and others which show the delay to have been brought about by external influences—by inappropriate modes of living, faulty education, etc. But it is oftener the consequence of a lymphatic temperament, of a scrofulous and weakly constitution, in which vitality is below a healthy standard. The retardation of this natural process will, in these instances, aggravate the condition of the already suffering individual.

When the non-appearance of the menses is due to the absence of the ovaries, or of the womb, the changes in the characteristics of the girl are rather masculine than feminine—in coarseness of features, skin, voice, etc. Such instances, although extremely rare, have been recorded.

When menstruation is delayed by constitutional or accidental causes, the girl retains all her feminine attributes, but looks immature and awkward; she may experience, monthly, the premonitory symptoms, and yet menstruation not appear. Pain in the back and the groins, general lassitude, deranged appetite, nausea, headache, may be present for two or three days, then disappear, and return at about the same date, the next month.

In girls inclined to consumption this delay is very significant; it indicates so little vitality, such a morbid state of the system, as to disable some of her most important organs; it is a condition which portends mischief for the future, and which, when accompanied by a cough, short breathing, hoarseness, sore throat, or pains in the chest, may be taken as something for immediate and careful attention.

HYGIENIC TREATMENT.

The treatment should be simply hygienic, unless the general health is so impaired as to require a medical one. For all amenorrhœa, but particularly for that class induced by a scrofulous constitution or by a lymphatic temperament, a regimen that is calculated to give tone to the general system is all that is needed. The girl should be taken from school, from all debilitating influences, such as bad air and poor diet, from the exciting and exhausting scenes of city life, and sent to the country, to the mountains or sea-shore, to breathe pure air, rich in oxygen; take daily exercise and have sunshine and nourishing food. A season of this kind has brought many an enfeebled girl to a state of vigor and health which would before have seemed almost impossible.

Beware of forcing-medicines; of drugs that have been known to perform "miracles." Do not forget that amenorrhœa is not in itself a disease, but the symptom of a disease; that the administering a drug to force menstruation, would, in such a case, be as logical as the attempt to prevent the fall of a house by removing the bricks that crumble from it. Moreover, at that time, when the system labors under some unknown difficulty, a drug may greatly add to the complication.

SUPPRESSION.

Before treating of this topic it may be necessary to explain the pathological difference between *suppression* and *retention*. "Suppression" is the failure of nature to perform the process of menstruation; while in "retention" nature has performed the process, but for some reason, probably mechanical, the blood is not permitted to flow out, and is arrested within the chamber of the uterus. As an illustration, suppose a reservoir from which water is expected to flow: at a given time, you open the spigot and no water comes. You at once inquire, Where is the obstacle? You examine the reservoir and find no water in it; the usual stream has failed to feed it; *it is a case of suppression.*

But if, on examining into the cause of the non-appearance of water, you find the reservoir is full, you come to the conclusion that, the stream having supplied it, the obstruction is in the spigot; *it is a case of retention.*

The failure of an organ to perform its functions should not properly be regarded as a distinct malady, requiring special treatment; but in view of the importance of the function of menstruation, and the quantity of fluid excreted, Suppression may become the immediate cause of grave disease, and therefore requires particular attention.

The causes of suppression may be divided into *pre-disposing* and *accidental*. The pre-disposing causes depend upon the constitution of the individual, her organization of the uterine organs, temperament, and degree of sensibility of the genital organs. When a pre-disposition exists, immediate causes will act as auxiliaries in producing suppression, and these are: poor nourishment, the use of acid beverages, a sedentary life, too much sleep, unhealthy habitations, over-work, late hours, or the use of articles of a stimulating nature, as rich viands, aromatic substances, and alcoholic fluids; also, moral affections, such as sadness, grief, disappointment, etc.; debilitating maladies anterior to the suppression, such as hemorrhages and other excessive evacuations; the use of astringent medicines, and the repression of the calls of nature.

Among the *accidental* causes we find sudden exposure to cold and humid air, when the body is over-heated; partial or general immersion of the body into cold water, icy cold drinks, abstraction of blood, either professionally or accidentally; a wound, a blow, a burn, a fall, an excessive pain, a strong odor, a great mental shock, powerful drugs, an irritated stomach.

Either of these accidental causes, occurring at a time when menstruation should appear, might induce suppression. The maladies following a suppression from accidental causes are generally acute, such as fevers, inflammations, etc.; while those resulting from simple pre-disposing causes are likely to be gradual, chronic, but progressive.

The liability to this suppression varies in different women; those who are pre-disposed to it through an inherited idiosyncrasy, or who have incurred the habit, have been subjected to a suppression by the slightest cause, such as even the change of linen; while those who are not so pre-disposed have exposed themselves to all the above mentioned causes with impunity.

Suppression is generally attended by the following symptoms: heat, heaviness or pain at the small of the back, extending sometimes to the end of the spine, and to the groins. The last vertebra may be so sore as to make it impossible to retain a sitting posture. Not unfrequently the pains of the abdomen are short and shooting, attended by swelling and tightness; the breasts also, sympathetically affected, become tumified and painful, and yield a white fluid, often mistaken for milk. When the suppression is long continued, the whole system responds to the unnatural condition; the appetite is lost, or replaced by a desire to eat strange things; the irritable stomach rejects food, or is troubled by nausea; the heart, oppressed, is subject to palpitations; the head is full and heavy, and oftentimes excruciatingly painful; the ears ring with strange sounds; the intestines, in their turn, are irritated, producing diarrhœa or dysentery; the bladder, the next neighbor to the womb, shares in the general derangement, causing frequent and difficult urinations.

This condition finally induces general lassitude, sadness or malaise. Women thus affected give external evidence of their condition by their faces becoming pale and puffed, their flesh flabby, their movements languid; they yield easily to moral influences, and become morose or melancholy. This debilitated and depraved condition makes them prone to neuralgia, hysteria, hypochondria, glandular enlargements, eruptions of the skin, etc.; to dropsical effusions, partial or general, manifested in the eye-lids, in the feet, in the pleura—the membrane around the lungs, in the pericardium around the heart, or in the entire skin surrounding the body.

The severest symptoms are more liable to occur when the suppression is sudden, and in subjects of lymphatic temperament; also in those of nervous and sanguine temperament, who have been subject to profuse menstrual discharge before the accidental suppression.

The indispositions that follow suppressions generally diminish in intensity, or entirely disappear, during the intervals between the menstruating periods, but are prone to increase during the time that menstruation should appear.

The effect of suppression depends upon its causes and duration. When induced by slight causes their removal is sufficient for the restoration of normal menstruation. Again, it sometimes happens that the woman's system adapts itself to a continued suppression without incurring serious consequences.

Yet the consequences are generally serious, and if continued beyond what might be reasonably expected from an accidental cause, medical counsel should be secured without delay.

Nature, oppressed by the retention of a fluid that should be monthly eliminated by the womb, attempts other means to obtain relief; thus hemorrhages of the nose, of the lungs, of the hemorrhoidal veins, have periodically occurred in place of the more natural process of menstruation; such hemorrhages are called "vicarious."

Menstruation is suspended during pregnancy of course. (See author's *Maternity*.) The exceptions to this rule are so few and rare as to need no special mention here.

SELF EXAMINATION.

One cannot look at the array of symptoms mentioned to describe this disease without being appalled at the possible consequences of suppressed menstruation. We trust that the description will not discourage the reader from examining for herself the condition in which she may be; on the contrary, we hope that her interest has been awakened in a subject the knowledge of which may give her health, and protect her from disease. She should commence her inquiry by contrasting her former condition with the present one, and ask: "Am I of a scrofulous or lymphatic temperament? was my usual condition a feeble, languid, or torpid one? was my appetite good, and my digestion normal? was my menstruation regular and sufficient? have I had any serious illness of the stomach, lungs, bowels, or spine? has anything ever occurred to cause me poignant grief or mental shock? is my disease traceable to any moral or physical affection?" Supposing her to be able to answer No, to these queries, the question still arises: What suppressed the menses? Did they stop suddenly; or fail to come when expected? Allowing an affirmative answer to either of the last, her endeavor should then be to discover the cause. Has she had a fright? Is she nursing a grief or disappointment, has she exposed herself to wet, or to sudden cold, has she over-worked, etc.? (See "Immediate causes.") Satisfied with her own answers to these, then the question should arise in her mind: What will be the probable result of this suppression? The answer will depend upon whether the suppression is accidental or habitual. If *accidental*, menstruation may return when due without any ill consequence; if *habitual*, the consequence may be very serious.

Amenorrhœa is *not* necessarily a grave malady, unless complicated with great constitutional disturbance, or dependent upon some remote disease; isolated and recent, it may prove but a delay. Having taken all the above into consideration, having made a satisfactory examination of her own condition and determined the causes of the suppression, the patient may be able to decide whether it is in her power to obviate the causes and remedy the evil, or whether she should give herself up to the better judgment of a medical counselor.

HYGIENIC TREATMENT.

The prescription of drugs should be left to the medical attendant, who alone is capable of prescribing for each individual case, every one having a decided individuality. Especial caution must be here given against the use of menstrual *nostrums* loudly proclaimed to "do the business" at short notice without failure. It is particularly against newspaper advertisements of miraculous cures that we warn the patient. Respectable physicians never advertise their treatment or themselves. The quack's circular may describe your case precisely, because such cases are common and well described in books; that description which has attracted your attention, which has been taken from estimable authors, is the trap into which he desires you to fall. If you need medicine, apply to a physician well known not only for skill but integrity. Again, you should be cautioned against any "panacea" of old women; however honorable their intention, they are not able to prescribe for your case. Forcing-medicines may prove most disastrous; in forcing the womb to menstruate, inflammations, already existing, may be so aggravated as to put life in danger.

A properly regulated regimen will not only prevent amenorrhœa, but in many instances cure it.

Simple cases of suppression, originally depending upon debility and a lymphatic temperament, and occasioned by poor nourishment, ill-ventilated and damp apartments, should be treated with a generous diet of roasted or broiled meats, wines, etc.; the patient should practice dry frictions over the body, dress warmly, and take moderate exerercise. A trip to the mountains or to the sea-shore, a few rides on horseback, a wholesome fortifying diet, have often been enough to bring roses to the pallid cheeks of girls. In another case, if the subject is of a strong sanguine temperament, nourishment should be of the lightest kind, beverages of water, and rest imperative.

It should be remembered that the tendency of menstruation is to reappear; that in due time nature makes the effort to re-establish it; it is *then*, therefore, that the means to assist it should be employed, that foot and hip-baths of hot water are particularly efficient.

Suppression induced by exposure to cold or dampness, or by checked perspiration, should be treated with warm drinks while in bed, for the purpose of restoring the action of the skin. When caused by mental impressions, as anger, grief, fright, jealousy, etc., a general warm bath will quiet the nervous system, and establish harmony between the relative functions of the mind and the bodily organs.

If the suppression is accompanied by an excess of pain, warm hip-baths, local application of hop poultices, hot, will be very useful. When suppression resists all treatment, a change of climate, a long journey by sea, may prove efficacious.

When the condition is dependent upon moral causes, great sagacity will be required on the part of the parents and the medical attendant, for as long as that state exists all the drugs of the pharmacy will be used in vain; but journeys, change of scene or surroundings, pleasurable distractions will be the only means of restoring health to the patient.

The use of spring-waters (particularly the ferruginous) and sea-baths may, however, prove of great benefit to persons of lymphatic temperament.

In cases where mental exaltation in affairs of love is the cause of the suppression, marriage has proved permanently curative.

Such is the treatment in all simple cases; when complications with remote maladies of a serious nature exist, the case should be referred to a physician.

RETENTION.

We come now to consider cases of RETENTION. The pathological difference between retention and suppression has been described above. The ovaries and the uterus have performed their functions, but the blood exuded within the chamber of the womb finds no exit. This is a dangerous and painful malady, and if no means are ready at hand to relieve the womb of the blood collected therein, even life may be put in danger.

The causes that may induce such retention are various and peculiar; they may be organic, as, when the mouth of the womb is closed by adhesions, and when the hymen is imperforated; instances are on record where the vagina was even found entirely absent. Such cases of adhesion however, are exceedingly rare, but may be induced by repeated inflammation of those organs, and by the treatment with caustics. When the closure is complete, there can be no flow whatever; but when incomplete, the flow is scanty, slow, difficult and painful.

Retention however, is generally induced by spasmodic closure of the womb, which yields easily to proper treatment. When the entire menstrual fluid is retained, the womb becomes distended and very painful; the distension increases every month, until, if not removed, it may burst the womb itself. Flexions of the womb, (that is, the womb bending upon itself,) the pressure of a polypus, or of any tumor, may induce complete or partial retention.

The symptoms of retention are like those of painful menstruation, but greatly intensified; the pains in the lower part of the abdomen are intensely severe and acute; they are of a forcing, bearing-down nature, pressing towards the bladder, causing frequent and difficult urinations. Under this great stress the nervous system becomes excited, producing chills, headache, hysteria, and sometimes even convulsions.

It is evident that the nature of retention is so grave, that none but a skillful physician is qualified to treat it. When retention is the consequence of spasmodic closure of the neck of the womb, and the patient has been so informed by her physician, very hot hip-baths, or a drink of warm water, such as would produce vomiting, will relax the muscular fibers, and give prompt relief to the patient.

It is scarcely needful to say more regarding this subject, as every case requires the most thorough investigation, and the most careful treatment of a physician.

CHLOROSIS (" *Green Sickness.*")

Chlorosis is not properly a disease of the generative organs of woman, and would have no place in this volume were it not that amenorrhœa is invariably connected with it. It is a disorder characterized by intense paleness of the skin, lips, and the lining membrane of the eye-lids; it is a paleness having a greenish hue, (from which the disease takes its name); at times the color is yellow, when it is often mistaken for jaundice. The noticeable and peculiar paleness of the lips and of the membrane over the eye-ball are almost infallible evidence of chlorosis.

Pathologically, the disease is distinguished by a lack of red globules in the blood, which seems as if turned to water; and the transfusion of that water through the veins into the cellular tissue causes dropsy of the face, of the feet, or of the whole body; it is this dropsica' condition that gives the "puffy" appearance. This disease, when continued, gradually weakens the patient, whose system under the general anæmia becomes deranged. The appetite is lost or perverted to a desire for strange things, such as slate-pencils, chalk, dirt, salt, charcoal, pepper, vinegar, pickles, lemon juice, etc.; then a sensation of weight oppresses the stomach, digestion is retarded, giving rise to evolution and eructation of gas; the respiration becomes labored, and palpitations of the heart are induced by the slightest exercise or mental excitement. This low condition predisposes the patient to neuralgia, which may affect the head, the neck, the eyes, the back, or any part of the body.

Chlorosis consists, essentially, of a watery state of the blood; the red globules being wanting, death-like pallor and weakness ensue, the menstrual and fecal discharges are suppressed. It is useless to discuss here the various theories advanced by pathologists regarding the exact nature of this disease; they disagree on this point, but concur that the almost constant absence of menstruation during the course of the disease is not the cause, but the consequence.

Chlorosis generally occurs at puberty, just before menstruating, although both married women and those who have menstruated have been affected by it.

A young girl in excellent health and color suddenly loses the roses of her cheeks, becomes intensely pale, loses her vitality, is tormented by notions and apprehensions; her cherry lips and the white of her eyes become greenish white. Soon her stomach shows irritability, refuses food or tolerates it with difficulty. Daily she grows weaker and more nervous, sleeps little and has frightful dreams. Now and then she complains of neuralgic pains in various parts of the body; she is moody, sensitive, hysterical. Spasms, convulsions, St. Vitus's Dance, epilepsy, may overtake her; the menses are suppressed, but she will probably be troubled with bleeding from the nose, of watery blood. Her heart jumps at the slightest cause; her breathing is oppressed. She has chlorosis.

This disease is generally curable, particularly when it does not occur in women of vitiated constitutions, and who have not been exposed for a considerable time to deprivation of healthy diet and pure, dry air. The danger of this malady lies in the organic diseases that may follow. Some of which are: valvular disease of the heart, dropsy, paralysis, hœmorrhages, consumption. The appearance or reappearance of the menses is the most reliable sign of the return of strength and health, and of a complete recovery.

The causes that predispose to this affection are strong mental emotions, fright, love, sexual excitement, masturbation, insufficiency or inferiority of food; residence in damp, close, unlighted, unventilated localities.

HYGIENIC TREATMENT.

A preventive regimen requires nutritious diet. If the girl has no desire for fresh meats she may relish salted or smoked beef and fish, codfish, mackerel, herring, oysters, clams, crabs, dried or smoked beef or ham. Brown, or rye bread, and good broths are excellent, and often acceptable; indeed, the stomach needs to be indulged to the last degree. Claret wine, ferruginous waters, are beneficial; but, above all, mountain air, sea shore, sea-journeys, open-air exercise, dry and well-ventilated apartments, will be more conducive to the restoration of her health than anything else.

CHAPTER IV.

MENORRHAGIA (EXCESSIVE MENSTRUATION).

THIS consists in either *too profuse*, *too prolonged*, or *too frequent* menstruation.

The quantity of blood discharged at one menstrual crisis varies in different women, and sometimes in the same subject; yet every woman has a knowledge of her average of flow, either as regards quantity or duration. (See Chapter XI., Part I., on "Philosophy and Physiology of Menstruation.") When she discharges more in the same length of time; when her periodical flow is prolonged beyond her usual time; when it recurs oftener than once a month, and the amount passed away in the month's cycle is beyond the usual quantity expected from the individual, the woman is said to be afflicted with *Menorrhagia*.

Naturally woman menstruates once every four weeks, allowing a few exceptions who menstruate oftener without ill consequences; the quantity lost each time is estimated to be about six ounces; the usual duration four or five days. Suppose, then, a girl to menstruate twice a month, each time a regular quantity; another, to menstruate in a regular manner as to periodicity and length of time, but secreting a much larger quantity; another, flowing not immoderately but continuously for ten or twelve days: it becomes evident that in each and every such case the loss of blood is in excess of the usual habit, requiring attention and treatment lest the general health become seriously affected from the unwonted drain.

In menorrhagia the quantity must be an *unusual* one for the person complaining, as some young women may discharge ten or twelve ounces regularly and yet be in a normal condition; while in others a discharge of eight or ten ounces would be considered unusually superabundant, and therefore menorrhagic. The normal individual quantity depends upon individual constitution and temperament, as already explained in the chapter on the "Physiology of Menstruation." There are women also who naturally menstruate twice a month, or once in three weeks, but in quantities that, if added together, do not yield a total in excess of what is natural and usual; hence not menorrhagic.

An inordinate flow occurs generally in women of sanguine temperament, whose hearts' impulse is strong and whose circulation is free. This temperament predisposes to determination of blood, and it is therefore reasonable to suppose that the womb, under the seasonable stimulus, may receive and discharge an abundant quantity of menstrual fluid. It is seldom, however, that an *excessive* flow occurs, unless a debilitating cause exists. The sanguine temperament, exuberant in action, may overreach its limits of vital powers, and terminate in debility.

Again, where the passions are strong and exposed to over-excitation, reflex action might determine blood to the generative organs and induce congestions that nature relieves by a profuse menstruation.

Luxury, indolence and indulgence enervate the human

system, however strong; and, therefore, it not seldom happens that a person of sanguine temperament is comparatively weaker than another who manifests less exuberance of constitutional vitality. Some morbid stimulus has exhausted the vital powers, destroyed the tone of tissues, induced anæmia, and relaxed the walls of the womb, on account of which the blood flows without restraint. Therefore, although a woman of sanguine temperament may be expected to discharge a larger quantity of menstrual fluid than one of a lymphatic temperament, yet, when the quantity is increased much beyond the habitual flow, a cause for the abnormal condition must exist which should be investigated and removed.

Menorrhagia is common also among women of nervous, irritable temper; in those who are corpulent and of indolent habits, and those who live in hot climates or who occupy rooms having a high temperature; it is also an hereditary predisposition; and, whatever its source, it is generally aggravated during the summer season.

Beside the constitutional tendency, there are *accidental causes* which may induce immoderate menstruation, among which are the following: exposure to excessive heat or cold; violent exercise, particularly on horseback and over rough roads; abuse of medicines intended to force menstruation; abuse of stimulants and of the pleasures of the table; a fall; lifting weights; mental excitement, such as fright, anger, jealousy, love, ambition, etc.

Reliable authorities insist that menorrhagia is invariably due to irritation and inflammation of the womb or ovaries; that the disease is local and not constitutional; that the morbid sensitiveness, the weakness, the moral and mental disturbances present in this disease are not causes, but effects of the excessive loss of vital fluid and of the uterine irritation communicated by reflex action. Others, quite as reliable, honestly differ from the above, and assert that in many instances this malady is induced, not by local, but by constitutional causes. We are of the opinion of the latter, and advise the patient to consult the medical man, who, upon due investigation, will determine the causes affecting the special case brought to his notice.

Hemorrhage should not be confounded with *menorrhagia*, although the latter implies a hemorrhage, both meaning a flow of blood: but menorrhagia is associated with menstruation, while simple hemorrhage is not. In other words, menorrhagia is either a too profuse, too prolonged, or too rapid recurrence of the *menstrual* flow; while hemorrhage may occur at any time from the womb, the lungs, etc., and from accidental causes. A hemorrhage of the womb may be a consequence of a blow, the application of a sharp instrument, pregnancy, labor, or abortion; also the presence in the womb of a tumor or some destructive disease as ulceration or cancer; it obeys no law of periodicity, but occurs at irregular periods and continues as long as the local lesion remains unchecked by active treatment; and while it may be slight and harmless, it may also be profuse and immediately dangerous. Menorrhagia may, in being prolonged and repeated, slowly deplete a person of blood, and thus withdraw so much of the vital force as to put life in peril; but the process will be gradual, and afford time for repair, for treatment, and for protection against collapse.

Menorrhagia may be *active* or *passive*, even *nervous* or *spasmodic*. The active kind results from an excess, the passive from a deficiency, of vitality. In the first, plethora is made apparent by the animated face, the strong, full pulse, the highly colored cheeks, the brilliant eyes; also by a liability to congestive headaches, feelings of general heat, rush of blood to the head, heaviness at the back of the stomach, heat and itching of the vagina. The second is marked by the lymphatic appearance and by paleness, anæmia, puffiness, indigestion, want of appetite, cravings for strange things, general debility, slow and weak pulse. The flow of the former will be of clear red blood, as if coming from a cut, while that of the latter is of lightly colored, watery blood.

In a plethoric woman, an active flow may prove beneficial, and remove all the unpleasant feelings she complained of before its occurence; but in a lymphatic, debilitated woman, even a passive flow will augment her weakness, and if continued induce fainting, dropsy, obscuration of vision, buzzing in the ears, dizziness, palpitation of the heart, discoloration of the skin, hysteria and possibly convulsions.

The above should be sufficient to warn women that menorrhagia may be so complicated and grave as to require the counsel of the most skillful physician. A general and local examination should be made, so that no false assurance should lead the patient into fatal indifference, or add a useless anxiety to the mental burden already oppressing her.

HYGIENIC TREATMENT.

The hygienic treatment will depend upon constitution and temperament. In sanguine temperaments excited by mental causes, quiet, rest, light and unstimulating food should be enjoined; the moral disturbances removed. Entire change from the locality, the scenes and the companionship that excited the mind and the senses will prove highly beneficial. If mental labor, in the transaction of business, in the attainment of professional or literary success, in study, in gratifying ambition or pride, has been the cause, a complete remission or intermission of those pursuits will be necessary. The mind must rest adequately to its labor, else a nervous exhaustion will follow, that will lower the vital powers of every organ of the body. A vegetable diet and acidulated beverages, lessening the red globules of the blood and diminishing the over-action of the heart, will be found particularly useful in plethoric persons.

When menorrhagia is induced by anæmia, debility, constitutional or otherwise, or in consequence of malarial fevers or of diseases of long standing, the regimen recommended in amenorrhœa will be applicable to it. Moderately cold hip or entire baths are generally invigorating to the feeble, particularly if quickly taken and followed by brisk frictions They are useful also to women of sanguine temperament, who may remain longer in the cold bath, thus permitting abstraction of heat. In either case, care should be taken not to plunge into a cold bath immediately before, during, or immediately after menstruation.

Menorrhagia depending upon inflammatory or structural diseases of the womb requires such positive and specific treatment as would be out of place in a volume of this character, and it is therefore properly referred to the care of the physician, who should be made acquainted with every detail connected with the case to enable him to prescribe with intelligence and skill.

CHAPTER V.

DYSMENORRHŒA (PAINFUL MENSTRUATION).

THE suffering connected with this disorder is of the most intense and acute character; and reflecting that a girl thus affected is monthly condemned to its recurrence, each time prostrating her on a bed of agony, the hardest heart would deplore her destiny.

But, probably, only the sufferer herself can realize that three or four days of writhing, wringing, cutting abdominal pains, returning once a month, is a penalty too severe, too cruel to be inflicted on a human being were it even intended as a retribution for crime; and when the torture is inflicted on an innocent girl, heart and mind rebel against the castigation. Yet thousands of unmarried women periodically bear this torture, smiling during the short intervals of ease that come between the spasms that seem to rend them. There is a pain-enduring capacity in woman that certainly man knows not of; in the throes of labor she smiles in anticipation of gladness, in the racking pains of dysmenorrhœa she only prays for the hour of relief. It is that struggle between the moral and the physical from which woman comes out a heroine.

But it is on this very account that our best efforts and greatest sympathy should be engaged in protecting and relieving her from such terrible fate It is to be regretted that often the most energetic means have failed to relieve; this failure is, however, generally due to a misconception of the origin and cause of the difficulty, and must be incurred whenever the trouble is treated as an independent difficulty while it is but a symptom of a deeper and remote disease.

Dysmenorrhœa is due very generally to inflammation or congestion of the ovaries or womb, yet it may be of neuralgic or rheumatic origin, or due to nervous irritability of the womb, the spasmodic strictures of its mouth interfering with a free flow of the menstrual fluid, causing partial retention and giving time to the blood to coagulate, each coagulation having to be thrust out by the contractile force of th womb. Menstruation suddenly suppressed by any accidental cause may become very painful and assume the form of dysmenorrhœa. During a high state of inflammation plastic lymph is sometimes exuded in the womb, organizing a pseudo-membrane like that of diphtheria or croup in the throat, passing off entire or in shreds, with the keenest pain. This has been styled "membranous dysmenorrhœa."

Malposition or flexion of the womb, tumors, or any mechanical obstruction may render menstruation difficult and painful.

Women of sanguine and nervous temperament are predisposed to dysmenorrhœa, particularly when they indulge in indolence, rich food, ardent spirits, wines, the pleasures of the senses; or are exposed to mental impressions of an exciting character.

This disease affects especially unmarried women, and marriage has often cured the disorder.

The *direct* or *accidental* causes are manifold, for almost any shock to the system may induce dysmenorrhœa in subjects predisposed to it; but moral disturbances, sudden transitions from heat to cold, or *vice versa*, any morbid affection of other organs, are pre-eminent causes of dysmenorrhœa.

The *symptoms* are of a very violent character; they generally commence three or four days before menstruation, increasing in intensity until the flux is fairly established; the erect posture aggravates them. They are as follows: pain in the back extending to the groins, and in the abdomen over the whole region of the womb as high as the navel, sometimes radiating down to the thighs. The pains gradually assume the spasmodic and colicky form, until they become unbearable; the blood flows by drops and sometimes in little clots, or is accompanied by membranous shreds. In highly nervous temperaments the excitement is so great as to induce hysteria and even convulsions. Under this excitability of the generative organs the breasts swell and become painful; gases are evolved in the abdomen, and a sensation of heat is felt in the vagina and the soft parts. The bladder sympathizes and urine is passed often, but with difficulty and a sensation of scalding. These symptoms may be premonitory and disappear as quickly as the flux appears; but more often, if the flow is not free, they increase for twenty or thirty hours, and may not end till the end of the discharge. The flow is generally scanty, but may be profuse; in the latter case, however, intermissions of suppression occur, during which the pains return with the usual severity; this is especially the case in women of highly nervous organization, susceptible to every impression. Generally a free flow relieves the pains as if by magic. In very young girls the womb may not be sufficiently developed, in which case the disorder cannot be expected to be cured until that organ is grown to adequate proportions. The natural cavity of the womb is very small, not retaining more than fifteen or twenty drops of the fluid, so that it may be easily comprehended that a very small quantity of blood may cause such distention as to induce excruciating pain.

When dysmenorrhœa recurs for many months and becomes habitual it may gradually induce such disorganizations of the womb as to cause it to become permanently diseased, unless properly treated.

Authors have differed regarding the causes of dysmenorrhœa; we will quote one, who says: "Ordinarily the primary and true seat of the morbid process, known as painful menstruation, is to be sought for in the highly irritated, congested, or inflamed condition of one or both ovaries, which condition is induced under a great variety of circumstances: from application of cold, from falls upon the knees or sacrum, from horseback riding, dancing, or long, fatiguing walks just previous to, during or immediately after, the menstrual flow, from great muscular effort, as the lifting of heavy weights, from tight dresses, corsets, and the various bands and strings around the waist, preventing a free returning of the blood from the pelvis; from retention or suppression of the catamenia [menses], from gouty or rheumatic habit, from solitary practices, etc.;" to which we add: from constipation, from mental excitement (particularly of the affections), from anger, fear, disappointment.

To give a clearer view of this trouble in all its phases we will divide it into classes, and give the principal characteristic of each; we hope thus to enable the unprofessional reader to discern its several forms.

Simple Dysmenorrhœa. This is an uncomplicated form of the disorder, called "nervous" or "neuralgic." It is due to the morbid sensitiveness of the uterus or ovaries and aggravated by mental excitement, exposure to heat or cold, over-fatigue, rheumatism, overloading the stomach, constipation, etc. Nervous-sanguine temperaments, girls subject to neuralgic or rheumatic affections, are more liable to it. The distinctive symptoms are found in the great sensitiveness of the uterine regions; the girl cannot be touched by the hand without an increase of pain, and even the weight of her clothing seems unbearable. At the approach of the menstrual period, sensations of fullness, weight and bearing down are felt at the vulva, and pains supervene which radiate to the bladder, the rectum and down the thighs. As the flow commences the pains become more intense and spasmodic, often amounting to actual cramps, and simulating labor pains. Women have been heard to exclaim, "I would rather give birth to a child than be subject monthly to these pains." Usually, after twelve or fifteen hours, when menstruation becomes fully established, the pains abate, passing gradually away, to the great relief of the patient; but it does often occur that they last during the whole course of menstruation. During the intervals, however, she is perfectly well, the parts not unnaturally sensitive, which is proof that there is no local inflammation. The suddenness of the attack, its severity and paroxysmal character, its recurrence month after month without affecting the general health, should be accepted as evidences that the case is one of irritability of the uterus, and of a neuralgic form.

Accidental Dysmenorrhœa. This is also one of the simplest forms that may occur occasionally from hygienic errors on the part of the woman immediately previous to, or during, menstruation. Overfatigue, excitement, exposure to cold may at such a time induce painful menstruation, which *does not recur at the following period.*

Congestive dysmenorrhœa is generally distinguished from the others by the clots which pass during menstruation. Congestion is a rush of blood to the womb, and may be compared to the rush of blood to the head causing apoplexy. The veins and arteries are engorged, causing all the pains of dysmenorrhœa with all the concomitant nervous symptoms which are very severe, but generally of short duration. Vomiting, convulsions, hysteria, may occur during the stage of congestion; but as soon as the blood flows sufficiently to relieve the overdistended vessels the symptoms disappear, and the patient is well.

Inflammatory Dysmenorrhœa. This is not a constitutional dysmenorrhœa, but the result of an inflammation of the womb and ovaries. It does not commence at puberty, like the constitutional, but occurs at any time in married, or unmarried women, when that morbid condition of the womb or ovaries exists. In this form the sufferings continue during the whole period of menstruation, leaving the region *tender even after it.* The whole system sympathizes with the local inflammation, and languor and anæmia follow, giving a general and continued evidence of physical deterioration. It is in this form of dysmenorrhœa that the *pseudo-membrane is formed*, passing out of the womb in shreds with excruciating pains. There may be inflammatory dysmenorrhœa without the formation of this membrane, but the presence of the membrane is always proof of inflammation. Inflammatory dysmenorrhœa is generally attended by *fever*.

Mechanical or physical dysmenorrhœa. This depends upon organic imperfection of the uterine neck, such as constriction; deformities of structure, or malposition of the womb; thickening of the lining membrane induced by previous and repeated inflammations; adhesions; tumors; and finally, closure of the vagina or imperforation of the hymen. The symptoms of this form do not differ in any high degree from the others, and it is therefore difficult to determine the form except by the close examination of the medical man. A tumor, if of any size, may be detected by the enlargement of the abdomen that does not subside after menstruation. The malposition of the womb may be suspected, if pain in the back, sensation of bearing down, desire to pass water often, and passing it with difficulty, or constant desire to evacuate the rectum without doing so, or when doing so passing a small, hard, compressed stool, *continue* to occur *during the intervals* between the menstruating periods. And the entire closure from imperforation of the hymen, or adhesions of the vagina or womb, may be prognosticated, if all the violent pains of periodical dysmenorrhœa occur, *without* any discharge of menstrual fluid.

Authors give many varieties of dysmenorrhœa and do not always agree as to its pathology, or in the classification; but the above may be sufficient to warn girls, that dysmenorrhœa may be or may result in formidable disease, and that, therefore, it needs their earnest efforts to prevent even the simplest forms; and in difficult and complicated cases, their good sense should enable them to conquer their aversion to calling upon the physician for advice and treatment.

HYGIENIC TREATMENT.

It must be evident even to the common reader that this disease, except in its simplest form, requires medical and surgical treatment; and there is no disease where the rules of hygiene should be more strictly observed than in this.

For young girls every means should be exercised that will assist in a proper and regular establishment of this function; hence, when this process begins with pain, they should be taken from school and all places or occupation of confinement, from exciting scenes, and from mental labor; the ambition to excel even in ordinary studies should be checked; their life should be vegetative. Attendance at balls and theatres should be strictly forbidden, and the diet be of the blandest character and in conformity with the temperament. (See "Temperament" and "Food.") And, above all, care should be taken that an evacuation of the bowels be obtained *every day*, constipation being not only an aggravation but often the sole cause of the disorder.

It is very common for girls to seek relief from the suffering in intoxication. This remark may seem extravagant, yet we have known girls to take two ounces of pure brandy or whiskey at one dose, and declare that

that was the only means by which to secure relief. This practice is dangerous—first, because if it is a case of inflammatory dysmenorrhœa, the stimulant aggravates the disease; secondly, if it is of the mechanical form of difficulty, the stimulus is useless; thirdly, the habit of drinking may be acquired. There is no doubt that in some instances, and particularly in the neuralgic or simple forms, stimulants relieve; yet it would be greatly to their advantage if women should confine their efforts during the intervals of ease to the observance of every care to prevent the recurrence of the disorder, and leave the active treatment to the physician.

Opiates are also resorted to for the relief of this painful trouble, which are no less dangerous than stimulants; and we dare assert, from our personal knowledge and that gathered from other physicians, that drunkenness and opium-eating in women are habits often contracted from the habitual recourse to these baneful "remedies" during the pains of dysmenorrhœa. We regret to say, moreover, that physicians have carelessly encouraged those habits, thoughtless of the disastrous results, when they should instead have studied their cases thoroughly or turned them over to more skillful professional brothers if their own ability failed them.

Moderation in all things, should be the rule of all women suffering from dysmenorrhœa. Rheumatic and neuralgic patients, as well as those of a lymphatic temperament, should dress warmly, and never be exposed to dampness or drafts of cold air; those of a sanguine temperament should make frequent use of cold baths, taking the precaution to follow them quickly by brisk and hard dry rubbing; but nervous and lymphatic temperaments will find the warm bath more conducive to their comfort. During the three or four days just preceding the menses the body should be kept at rest in a reclined position, and every night a hot hip-bath should be taken before retiring. During the access of pain or spasms hot hip-baths, application of hot poultices to the abdomen, hot applications to the feet, mucilaginous— such as hot decoctions of hops, marsh-mallow, chamomile, etc.,—and vaginal injections of warm water will afford relief. If the bowels are not free, they should be moved by warm enemas of water. No iced water, or very cold drinks of any kind, should be taken immediately before or during menstruation; a mouthful of cold water has in many instances brought back all the pains that had been relieved by proper treatment.

CHAPTER VI.

LEUCORRHŒA ("WHITES.")

THIS disease, although not dangerous to life, is one of great discomfort and general debility. It consists of a flow of mucus from the genital organs, which varies according to the constitutional disturbance, and the locality and extent of the inflammation, being at times white (from which it takes its name), again bluish, yellowish, or red with blood; at times inodorous, again fetid. The seat of the irritation or inflammation may be in the walls of the vagina, the neck of the womb, the lining membrane of the womb itself, or the fallopian tubes.

Leucorrhœa being a symptom of some constitutional disturbance rather than a disease, has been by medical men classified according to its original causes; but in a work intended for the lay rather than the professional reader, a pathological classification would rather burden than assist in the comprehension of its description. As a principal cause of leucorrhœa we must note the constitutional inheritance as found in lymphatic subjects, ill-developed and feeble, generally known from their want of muscular vigor, their pallid faces, soft flesh, weak digestion, morbid and melancholic tendencies. (See "Lymphatic Temperament.") Girls of such constitutions may manifest, even during infancy, leucorrhœal characteristics, probably excited by irritation induced by dentition, or by the presence of worms.

External causes predisposing to this malady are sometimes found in the water of certain mineral springs, in the use of new beer, unripe fruit, milk diet, tea, and *café-au-lait*.

This last article of diet has, by a French author, been declared a very common cause of leucorrhœa among French women, who make daily use of it; the same author asserting that in cases where women refrained from the use of that stimulant they were permanently cured of the annoying discharge. Local irrritations from the application of instruments, the wearing of pessaries, or solitary habits of a vicious character have been found to be sources of this disease.

Not unfrequently leucorrhœa is induced by the suppression of some other malady, as a cutaneous eruption, rheumatism, gout, the suppression of a hemorrhoidal flux, a diarrhœa, or the milk in nursing women; the healing of an old ulcer, the sudden check of a chronic cough.

Again, and more often, it is the result of exposure to either heat or cold, insufficient or excessive exercise, dampness of the atmosphere, wet feet and damp clothing, badly ventilated apartments, insufficiency of light, malaria, poor nourishment, prolonged warm baths, medicated injections, obstinate constipation, rough travelling, riding a hard-trotting horse, inflammation of the womb or ovaries, uterine displacements or ulceration, abortions, and drugs intended to force menstruation.

Fevers, and particularly miasmatic and scarlet fevers, measles, and smallpox often terminate in leucorrhœa, which is then called *critical*, and regarded as a favorable symptom.

Of all the infirmities that afflict woman, leucorrhœa is probably the most common; it affects women of all ages and of all classes, but particularly during the period of menstruation. It is, moreover, an intractable disease, difficult to cure, and one against which physicians have often exhausted their skill and patience in vain.

The probable reason for their failure may be that it has too often been treated as a disease *per se*, rather than as a symptom of disease. No intelligent person could attempt to treat an expectoration as a disease, and prognosticate that when the expectoration ceases the disease is cured. The vagina and uterus are lined by the same mucous membrane that lines the bronchial tubes, an excessive exudation from which would be an evidence of irritation or weakness. There is nothing extraordinary in leucorrhœa, for it is only the excess of a discharge that should always be present for the lubrication of the walls, that would otherwise adhere to each other.

The quality of the discharge may vary just as does the quality of a bronchial discharge, both being dependent upon constitutional and local condition.

And in consideration of the monthly excitement and congestion of the ovaries and uterus, it is not surprising that a debilitated condition of the general system, or other causes affecting the organs of generation, should often determine an irritation of the uterine and vaginal follicles, exciting them to exude an inordinate flow of mucus.

Precursory Symptoms of Leucorrhœa. Heavy pains in the lower part of the abdomen and the small of the back; distaste for articles of food; lassitude; itching of the private parts, which may be tumefied and painful. This condition may be attended by dryness of the skin, fever and sleeplessness. Finally, mucous fluid escapes the vagina, varying in color and thickness. As the disease progresses the above symptoms are present in an aggravated form.

Acute Leucorrhœa. This form may be distinguished from the chronic by its more severe but shorter course.

When acute, the itching of the vagina may be so violent as to be almost unbearable; the local irritation spreads to the surrounding parts and to the bladder, inducing a constant desire to urinate. Soon the characteristic discharge makes its appearance, accompanied by a sensation of heat and distension of the affected parts.

For two or three days this condition becomes more and more aggravated; the discharge increases, and from white it turns to either yellow or green; the inclination to urinate becomes frequent, and the urine scalds; the local inflammation grows more intense, the pain more severe and prolonged. In the course of eight or ten days the inflammatory symptoms yield, however; but the discharge is still on the increase, and becomes thicker and of a deeper color. In two or three days more, even these last symptoms abate, and the patient becomes conscious of great improvement. Finally, if no error is committed, in twenty or thirty days the patient gets entirely well. The course of this accidental leucorrhœa is therefore acute, severe, and short.

Chronic Leucorrhœa may be a continuance of an acute form in consequence of bad treatment; and its course then is very irregular, and its duration uncertain. In the chronic form the discharge is continuous, although in some instances it intermits; the acute inflammatory symptoms, such as the intolerable itching and the tumefaction of the parts, may not be present, or only in a slight degree; the pains are less, more bearable, and intermittent; the vagina less painful to the touch.

But this form, although not severe, slowly undermines the general health from its continuance; the stomach takes up the sympathy, loses desire for food, or bears it unkindly, rejecting it at the slightest provocation; digestion, thus impaired, adds to the general bad condition, manifested by weariness, paleness or puffiness of the face, and indifference to pleasure; the head partakes of the general anæmia, and dizziness, fainting and hysteria supervene; the pulse becomes small and slow, and the perspiration scanty.

The patient then is very susceptible to cold and to all mental impressions.

There is also a *transient* form of leucorrhœa which may occur either before or after menstruation; oftentimes induced by disordered stomach, but borne without much trouble or suffering, passing away with the adoption of a proper diet and the restoration of a good digestion.

Leucorrhœa seems to replace in some instances the menstrual flux.

It has happened that instead of the menses a certain quantity of white mucus has been excreted periodically and regularly every month, lasting four or five days and then disappearing.

Intermittent leucorrhœa, arising from mechanical causes, yields easily to proper and preventive treatment;

when, however, it is a result of feeble, lymphatic and scrofulous constitutions, or of long duration, it may baffle the best efforts of medical art.

The mode of life influences the tenacity of leucorrhœa. When long-continued it interferes with the regularity of menstruation, reducing its quantity and changing its quality; it may even prevent the establishment of the menstrual functions at puberty. When it has existed for a long time and is suddenly arrested the malady may be transferred to other organs, as the lungs, exposing them to pneumonia or to a development of consumption if the patient is scrofulous.

In cases where there is a relaxation of the tissue of the vagina or of the muscles supporting the womb, this constant humidity tends to relax still more those tissues, thus forming displacements and falling of the womb.

A disease of this character, depending upon so many different causes, and particularly upon hereditary and constitutional disturbances, apparently simple, amenable yet complicated, and fraught with danger, requires so much discrimination and clearness of judgment that it seems as if no one but the most competent physician should be allowed to examine and advise. Regarded, as it often is, as a light indisposition, too little attention is given to it, and the recommendation of incompetent persons too readily adopted; it is probably due to this fact that leucorrhœa has been allowed to go on from year to year, until it has sapped the very foundation of a woman's health, and reduced her to a state of chronic valetudinarianism, or sacrificed her to the fatal effects of such diseases as ulceration or cancer.

Hygienic treatment. The treatment of this disease

should consist in the strict observance of the rules of hygiene; for a regimen, adapted to the case, is truly of more importance than all the preparations of the pharmacopeia. The leucorrhœal tendency being more generally due to constitutional weakness than to any other cause, it follows that anything calculated to improve the general health should be pre-eminent in the treatment; therefore, the patient should be removed from all enervating influences, of school duties, or any other occupation, of heat, cold or dampness, and sent to the country, where the atmosphere is pure and bracing. Her nourishment, with due regard to her capacity, should be generous, of digestible meats not overdone; Bordeaux, Rhine, Madeira, Port or Sherry wine, used with discretion, may be added to her dietary. She should take regular and systematic exercise in the open air, but proportionate to her strength, never beyond it; the exercise should be gradually increased, until she can walk three or four miles a day without prostration. She should not lift, nor carry weights, nor practice cooking by hot stoves. She should keep her skin in moderate perspiration by warm clothing, careful, however, not to expose herself to draughts of cold air. She should shun the ball-room, late suppers, and all scenes of excitement. She should not remain in wet shoes or garments; and when she has unavoidably exposed herself to getting wet, she should return home, walking rather than driving, immediately remove the wet articles, dry the skin by brisk friction, dress herself in dry garments, and move about until reaction is complete. Locally, she should keep the parts free from accumulations by daily ablutions and cleansing with castile soap and water.

CHAPTER VII.

HYSTERIA.

NAMES are seldom hazard expressions. That great philosopher, Shakespeare, makes Juliet say:

"What's in a name? that which we call a rose,
By any other name would smell as sweet."

In the extravagance of her love Juliet thought that but for his name, Romeo might have been an angel dropped from heaven for her delight; and that when she added, "Romeo, doff thy name," all that was human and historic would be thus removed, and he could be her own. But, unfortunately for her, the name was as much a part of Romeo as he was of his name, and the answer to this piece of philosophy was, that the name brought them both to a most tragical grave. So, there is a great deal in a name; and a man cannot "doff" his name any more than he can doff his skin. It is wonderful, in the study of the names of animals and things, to see how this philosophy has, from the earliest stages of human culture, been exercised in the selection of names! Character, occupation, station and rank were often known by the name of an individual. In the tongues of the Indian tribes, this method of naming men and things by their qualities has been constant, and in many instances the selection most appropriate and logical.

But in this case, hysteria would puzzle even an Indian; it is a name that reveals nothing of its history; it is the name of an organ, and not of a disease. Our ancient philosophers, ignorant of the pathology of this disease, located it in the womb, and then named it after that organ; *hysteria* meaning *uterus*. The only claim it has to that name is that, like the organ, the disease is peculiar to woman (this is denied, however, by later authors), and occurs only during the period of uterine development and menstrual evolution; seldom has it happened before puberty or after the close of menstrual life.

Hysteria is but little understood by people; to some it causes merriment, to others contempt; yet few are the maladies on account of which the patient deserves more sympathy and kindness. Just imagine a girl conscious of an inner power acting independently of herself, causing her to laugh when she should weep, and weep when she should laugh! Imagine one's command over oneself gone, or the body disobedient to the will! Imagine one talking immoderately when silence would become! Imagine an ecstasy when soberness would befit! Turning, twisting, writhing in extraordinary movements when modesty would forbid! Imagine one with a horrid pain shooting through the brain (a pain almost facetiously called "clavus hystericus," hysterical spike), being told by the physician that it is "nothing but hysteria"! Imagine a sensation as if a ball were rising in the throat suffocating one to death! Imagine convulsions, apparent death, with a pulse as even and regular as the tick of the most perfect clock! Yet, such is hysteria. Many pages might be filled with descriptions of its manifestations, so numerous and varied are they. Nevertheless, a person, nay, a girl, thus affected, receives no sympathy, because the disease does not kill! Many a tear has been shed over much less dangerous or troublesome affections; much sympathy been wasted where it was less needed! Still, no one can tell what hysteria is. The many names it has received from different pathologists only prove the ignorance existing regarding it. It is easily recognized by its manifestations, but its true origin is undiscovered.

When in ancient times the uterus was believed to be an animal, hysteria was believed to be the wanderings and vagaries of that animal within the body, as if in a frolic or carousal; later, when pathology became a science, some have attributed it to a morbid condition of the uterine nerves; others to a similar condition of stomach and bowels; others to congestions of lungs and heart; to spinal irritations, to cerebral excitement, to displacements of the womb, to inflammation, ulceration or irritability of the same, etc. It is a disease that has perplexed many a brilliant intellect; that has been explained only to have the explanation denied; it is useless to the purpose of this book, therefore, to examine into the various speculations regarding its origin; its immediate causes and manifestations will suffice, for everything else is uncertain.

Although this disorder is found among all classes of women, and in very rare instances in men, it is seldom found among the working class; its field of action is principally among that class who lead an indolent life, kept awake by the excitement of the imagination. Those peculiarly predisposed to hysteria are women of ardent temperament, pre-eminently sanguine and nervous; impressionable, lazy and feeble.

The causes that predispose to hysteria are: the effort of nature to establish menstruation at puberty; every thing calculated to irritate or inflame the generative organs; and delayed, suppressed, or painful menstruation. It must be acknowledged, in favor of the uterine theory, that a very large proportion of hysterical cases are associated with some derangement of the womb or the ovaries. Exposure to excessive heat or cold, winds, dampness, or the rays of the sun may produce an attack of hysteria; also violent exercise, fatigue, dancing, long vigils, irritating articles of diet, and, particularly, cheese, oysters, truffles, mushrooms, pepper, spices, etc.; extreme pressure of clothing; too frequent ablutions, particularly if warm; strong perfumes, rich food, and abuse of coffee, tea, wine or liquors; love, jealousy, disappointment, etc.

The *immediate* causes are: a fit of anger, a fright, a violent and sudden affliction, a reproach, improper conversations, the sight of a repulsive object, impressions from a tragical drama, somber music or an affecting story, humorous tales or plays exciting the risibles, contrariety, a sudden joy or the sudden appearance of an object of love or hatred, long and hopeless waiting, bad news, irritating applications to the skin, tickling, etc.

Hysteria (morally speaking) is infectious; if one girl falls into a fit of hysteria in the presence of other girls, some of the latter will very probably become affected in the same way. It is related of a boarding-school that it had to be closed, and the girls sent home, on account of the many cases that followed one which occurred in presence of the class.

Women predisposed to this affection present, generally, all the traits of a very impressionable nature; they are light, frivolous and opinionated; often capricious and irascible; of a humor inconstant and changeable. A trifle will cause them to pass from the most violent expression of joy, from an immoderate laugh, or from affectionate caresses, to sulkiness, sighs, tears and bitter reproaches; even to regret, self-accusation and melancholy.

It may be cruel to say of persons, whose illness makes them irresponsible, that they dissimulate; yet in hysteria this is frequently the case. The patient will often affect a malady that does not exist; and it is told of a lady who had kept her bed for many months, despite the remonstrances of friends and medical attendants, that the ruse of setting her bed on fire was resorted to; and that in her fright she flew out of bed and house, although she had always insisted that it would be death to her to move from it. She returned to her home and couch, but like other people, and in a natural condition, and from that time retired and rose regularly, without the slightest apprehension or sickness.

Again, other diseases, under the influence of hysteria, may be greatly exaggerated, irregular, and out of proportion to the real state of the affected organ. Hysterical coughs are so exaggerated as to lead one to suppose that pneumonia or phthisis is imminent; hysterical palpitations of the heart, of such violence as to make the patient believe that an organic disease is not only possible, but certain, the assurances of a skillful medical man to the contrary notwithstanding. Apprehension of pregnancy in married women predisposed to hysteria has so misled their intelligence that instances have come under our observation in which women, sensible in everything else, and who had experienced all the symptoms of pregnancy several times before, would insist that they were pregnant, and that they distinctly felt the motions of the child, when there was not a shadow of enlargement of the abdomen, and the womb was in a perfect state of quiescence. To induce the husband and attendants to believe with them they would resort to ruse and deception, and swallow sickening things to make themselves vomit. There is no end to the pranks of hysteria. Those subject to it are truly to be pitied; for their distress, whether feigned or true, is real to them. Generally, when accident or circumstances reveal their real condition, they become totally cured of that hallucination, and never refer to it again. It seems that the shock to the mind received by the humiliating discovery cures the mental obliquity of which they have been the victims. I knew a lady who feigned death. I was in Norfolk, Va., in June, 1865, when a well-known physician approached me, and related the case of a lady who was apparently dead, and who had been visited by several medical men who had all agreed that she was not dead but dying. This was her eighth day, however, and yet she was not a corpse; and the physician who met me was considerably exercised over the case. I said to him, "Go to her, bid her good-by, and tell her that, inasmuch as she will die in a few hours, you need not return. Do not go, but hide yourself so that you can watch her eyes without betraying your presence. If she winks, if her eyelids tremble, it is a case of hysteria; give her then a large injection [she would take nothing by the mouth, even a drop of water would remain unswallowed] of asafetida mixture." He did so; in half an hour she opened her eyes as from a deep sleep, spoke to her attendants as if nothing had been the matter with her, and, what is strange, never afterwards alluded to her case.

Catalepsy is apparent death; but although very rare, when it occurs it is invariably associated with hysteria. So, also, is that which is called *ecstasy* or *trance*. Hysterical convulsions may be mistaken for epilepsy; but in the latter there is *entire loss of consciousness*, while in the former there is not. The patient on emerging from an epileptic fit remembers absolutely nothing of what occurred during the paroxysm: not so during an hysterical fit—the loss of consciousness is never complete, and never occurs at the outset. There are other secondary points, such as foam, froth and blood issuing from the mouth of a patient during an epileptic fit, which never happen during an attack of hysteria, and other distinguishing characteristics which would not be of much use to the lay-reader.

The diseases that are often simulated by this one are: *Inflammation of the peritoneum* (the membrane covering and holding in place the organs within the abdomen). When acute pain in the abdomen, aggravated by the slightest pressure, is present, and is accompanied by hot skin, furred tongue and quick pulse, and the symptoms appear in a young female subject to irregularity of menstruation, the probability is that she is affected by hysteria, instead of that dangerous inflammation, *peritonitis*.

Pain in the side simulates *pleurisy*, diseases of the spleen or liver.

Partial *palsy* is also simulated by hysteria; but the hysterical paroxysms, and the sudden disappearance of the palsy after the paroxysm is over, should be an indication that the case is one of hysteria instead of true paralysis.

A sudden loss of voice, "aphonia," occurs in hysteria, leading the attendants to suppose an inflammation or disorganization of the larnyx: there are instances on record where surgeons have plunged the knife into the throat to relieve a supposed and fatal stricture, when in reality it was only an hysterical constriction, that could have been removed by simple remedies.

The breasts become tumefied, painful and tender, alarming the friends with the anticipation of cancer.

The hysterical cough is also common, and has led even medical attendants to believe in the approach of consumption or pneumonia; it is a loud, harsh, dry, spasmodic cough, more like a bark than a cough.

Hiccoughs and eructations, continuing unabated, have made people fear a deep-seated disease of the stomach.

The most common simulations are, however, pains in the joints and along the spine. These have kept women in bed for months, undergoing the most active old-fashioned treatment without improvement. It is in such cases that patients have believed it impossible for them to move, and retained the same position in bed, while they could have walked like any perfectly well person. Dr. Bright relates the case of a young lady who had been confined to her bed for nine months. If she attempted to move, she was thrown into a paroxysm of agitation and of great agony, particularly in the abdomen. She gave no evidence of disease whatsoever. She protested against getting up, declaring that it was impossible. Once he left her for a month, and when he returned he found her completely recovered; for, under a deep religious impression, she had abandoned her former hallucination, and had gone to work. It is in these cases that charlatans, Spiritualists, etc., raise people from the dead. They put the patient under the influence of a stronger impression, and she gets well. If they confined themselves to curing cases of hysteria, they might be of some use in society; but when they go on, wickedly pretending to cure organic diseases, they should be indicted.

Simple hysteria is quickly detected. Women called hysterical laugh or cry even immoderately, or commence with the former and end with the latter, for trivial causes that often would induce but a smile or a moment's soberness in others. During a play in which several persons are engaged, any unusual or general merriment will throw a girl into an immoderate and irrepressible fit of laughter, soon followed by long and deep sighs, which are only efforts to regain breath; she will then alternate the fits of laughter with fits of crying as if her heart would break, alarming some one with the idea of having given offense or pain. If this is not immediately checked by an extraordinary effort on her part, or her mind is not quickly diverted from the object that caused her to laugh, these fits become stronger; a sensation as if a ball were rising in her throat causes her to violently grasp her clothing to remove the object she fancies is choking her; she throws her limbs about and gets partially convulsed; her fingers tighten upon anything within reach, or are spread out like unarticulated sticks. She relaxes only to go in a little while into another paroxysm. During the remissions she moans, pities herself, bewails her fate; no one loves her, everyone is against her: she is inconsolable. She tells strange things; she repeats what she knows, whether it is injurious to others or to herself. Great secrets have thus been revealed, and quite as often exaggerated, and even invented. This condition may last but fifteen or twenty minutes, or may continue for hours, and even for days. One instance occurred in my practice in which a lady, who received a mental shock, fell into a hysterical fit, and for *twenty nights following* these fits recurred, commencing about nine or ten o'clock in the evening, and ending between four and five in the morning. During the day she was as well as usual, and it did not seem as if another attack were possible; yet, when evening came she became hilarious; her eyes sparkled, and she would become talkative and witty. These were the premonitory symptoms of another attack; these would only change in their order of appearance. Generally, while in this talkative state, during which her eyes were closed, she would relate amusing stories about herself, her mother, sisters, husband, doctor, and anyone else; or repeat Shakespeare by the page. Suddenly she would startle the attendants with a piercing shriek, exclaiming, "It is coming!" pressing her hands upon her temples. The clavus hystericus was upon her. From this she would pass into a convulsion, in which she would make a bow of her body backwards, so that pillows had to be put against the head-board of the bed lest her nose be broken. She would come out of a convulsion in two or three minutes, but in a moment more the "spike" would be driven through her temples again inducing the same alarming shrieks, to be followed by another similar convulsion. This would last sometimes an hour or two, when vomiting would supervene, and the body remain relaxed. This vomiting was, if possible, even more distressing than the previous condition; she would retch violently, vomiting but a little gluey mucus. In an hour or so this would pass off and she would fall into a semi-trance, answering questions, but following her own thoughts, and, with a smile on her face, would tell all the amusing incidents of her life, or those of persons present, or of absent friends. Finally, she would drop into a doze, from which she would come out refreshed and ready for her breakfast. This lady had had a similar attack years before. She was endowed with culture and a fine nervous organization, and was not an hysterical woman in the common acceptation of the term; she was brilliant in society, but always self-possessed. After twenty nights of such torture she came out of that condition slightly weakened, but with unimpaired health. Fifteen years have now passed, and although she has had her good share of human sorrows, hysteria has not again disturbed her.

A very noticeable fact in this disorder is, that although it may continue for days and months uninterruptedly, the digestive organs are seldom affected; the appetite continues unimpared, and the general system remains in a reasonably good condition.

It is a distressing malady but not a fatal one; no person has ever died of it unless complicated with some structural disease. It is probably due to this immunity from danger, and to the extraordinary and often foolish behavior of the afflicted ones, that people have learned to look upon this infirmity with indifference if not contempt.

TREATMENT.

As this is a disease peculiar to women of highly nervous temperament, of an exalted imagination, care should be taken to shield them from all causes predisposing to a development of hysteria. The more the brain is refined by education the more the susceptibility to this disorder is increased; and the fact that it is common among the refined class of the cities and exceedingly rare among the working women of the country is a proof that abundant and pure air, healthy exercise, and a brain untainted by the exciting scenes or temptations of city life are so conducive to that healthy and normal state of the nervous system as to secure exemption from this morbidity. Young girls at boarding-schools promiscuously associated with others, oftentimes of a depraved character, are in great danger. Let their minds remain pure; let them avoid conversations and literature of dubious character, shun everything of doubtful propriety, or they will incur imminent danger of becoming victims to a malady whose very name draws a smile of derision. It is conceded that love, and all its immoderate desires and disappointments, the morbid appetites of precocity and the depravity of the senses grown under improper sexual stimulus, lay the foundations for this disease, which, when acquired, will only leave the victim when nature has reached her limit and the body entered its season of decay.

In an issue of the New York *Tribune*, dated April 6th, 1875, we find the following pertinent remarks, which we gladly transfer here: "In fashionable, and would-be fashionable circles, the poor little infants are dragged to balls as soon as they are weaned, and converted into hot-pressed little men and women. The books furnished to them, the matinée entertainments provided for them, are all calculated to rouse adult passions and thoughts into abnormal, monstrous growth. There is no such thing as a nursery in the majority of American city homes. The children are left to the care of ignorant hired *bonnes* or Irish girls; they swarm in the halls of boarding-houses, or haunt the servants' rooms, trying to stretch their little brains to grasp the ideas and subjects which reach them there. When they have passed out of baby-hood, they are dismissed to schools, where they learn good or evil, as paid teachers or their companions choose. Let any one observe the groups of flaunting half-grown girls on their way to school in the cars, or the over-dressed coquettish misses sent out to parade the streets and display their clothes on a fine afternoon, and listen to their conversation, and he will not wonder at their escapades into marriage or a worse fate.

"It is not book-publishers who are to blame; it is not playwrights; it is not French *bonnes* or Irish nurses. They furnish what the public demands of them. The one thing needed to give us a generation of modest, chaste gentlewomen in our daughters, is—mothers. Mothers who know their business, and who do it; mothers who have the sense to see that there is a time in a young woman's life, as in a man's, when animal spirit, or excess of vitality, needs outlet; mothers who can guide their daughters through this strait in all innocence and purity, instead of subjecting them from their very birth to treatment which forces every impure element of their nature into unhealthy and obnoxious action."

Sir Benjamin Brodie's remarks on this point are not less pertinent: "You can render," he says, "no more essential service to the more affluent classes of society than by availing yourselves of every opportunity of explaining to those among them who are parents how much the ordinary system of education tends to engender the disposition of these diseases among their female children. If you would go further, so as to make them understand in what their error consists, what they ought to do, and what they ought to leave undone, you need only point out the difference between the plans usually pursued in the bringing up of the two sexes. The boys are sent at an early age to school, where a large portion of their time is passed in taking exercise in the open air; while their sisters are confined to heated rooms, taking little exercise out of doors, and often not at all, except in a carriage. The mind is over-educated at the expense of the physical structure; and, after all, with little advantage to the mind itself; for who can doubt that the principal object of this part of education ought to be not so much to fill the mind with knowledge as to train it to a right exercise of its intellectual and moral faculties; or that, other things being the same, this is more easily accomplished in those whose animal functions are preserved in a healthy state, than it is in others?"

The great majority of cases of hysteria depend upon some disorder of the generative function or from an exaggeration of the affections. In the former all that has been said regarding these functional disorders should be carefully noticed, and the regimen respectively applied as suggested, when it is evident that hysteria is a consequence of any one of them. In the latter, the parents should secure the confidence of their daughters, and apply such moral remedies as only a loving mother and father can suggest. The cause of the nervous derangement should be inquired into with care and circumspection, lest fear and suspicion be engendered in the girl, leading her to deceive. Change of locality, of habits and associations, may accomplish a permanent cure. What reasoning cannot effect, compulsion might; but the latter should never be resorted to until the former has been exhausted. Parents, above all, should never forget that they have been young, and that love, although devoted to an unworthy person, is neither unnatural nor a crime; that unreasonable opposition to or compulsory abandonment of her affection may throw the object of their solicitude into a much worse condition than if she had married the one she loved. Inoffensive watch should be kept over the habits of the girl predisposed to this malady, and in many instances it would be well for the mother to take the girl as her companion, and sharer of her room and bed. Let her have plenty of air, exercise, innocent and light amusements; but keep her from spectacular dramas, the ballets, impressive music, and the company of over-weening associates; from religious extravagances, and anything that would strongly impress the imagination.

The diet should be light and principally of vegetables; rich viands, wines, beer or liquors absolutely forbidden, except in special cases of anæmia.

During an attack, cold affusions are very beneficial, —sprinkling the face, or pouring a column of cold water from a pitcher on the head; the shock thus produced has often broken a spell instantly. Remove all tight dress-

HYSTERIA.

ing, place the patient on her bed, give her plenty of free air, and remove from the room every person calculated to keep up or increase the mental excitement. In long and continued paroxysms the physician should be in attendance.

CHAPTER VIII.

INFLAMMATION AND DISPLACEMENTS OF THE WOMB.

HAVING designed this book for the use of girls before they attain the state of nubility, we might claim that our task ends here; for the disorders that are common among girls, and that ordinarily lay the foundation for organic diseases of the womb when older or married, have already been treated of. But, inasmuch as these diseases are found, though rarely, even among unmarried women, who should enjoy perfect immunity from them if they attended faithfully to the hygienic rules adapted to their age and their condition, a résumé of the possible consequences of careless habits will be given in this chapter, with the view to warn them against excesses which, even if not immediately dangerous, are very likely to result in years of pain, feebleness, and suffering of various kinds, because sapping the health and strength of the characteristic organ of woman—the type of motherhood.

The womb up to the period of puberty is totally passive; has no functions to perform, except such as concern its own existence. It is not, therefore, then liable to inflammations or disorganizing diseases. But as soon as it reaches the stage of development for the preparation of the productive period, and becomes subject to a monthly orgasm, it is liable to all the diseases observed in the other organs of the economy. The more active an organ, the more liable to derangement, as may be noticed in the frequent diseases of the brain, of the lungs, of the stomach, bowels or liver, and the comparatively rare diseases of the spleen; hence, the ovaries and the womb, when in the dormant state, scarcely ever assume disease, but when actively engaged in the exercise of the functions peculiar to their organization are susceptible to all the influences surrounding them; nay, the extreme sensibility with which they are endowed, their peculiar irritability and physiological course, constitute a state of activity which dominates the entire physical life of woman. It is not, therefore, surprising that the womb, so much concerned in that physical life, should become deranged in its operations or disorganized by disease; indeed, it is marvelous that an organ subject to so many phases, to so many alterations, should maintain its integrity as often as it does. Supplied abundantly with vessels carrying blood, with nerves connecting it with nearly every other organ, it might be supposed that it would often be invaded by inflammations or nervous maladies, particularly when subjected to violence; but nature, having ranked it in the class of the noblest organs, has provided it with means of resistance which enable it to undergo the severest trials without perishing.

INFLAMMATION.

Inflammation of the womb is divided into the *acute* and the *chronic*. Acute inflammation of the womb, the ovaries or the vagina, is very rare amongst unmarried women. The distinguishing symptoms attending the acute form, however, are fever and severe local pain.

The pain in the region of the womb may be so acute as to render even the weight of the clothes unbearable; it extends to the back and even down the thighs; the parts are swollen, and sensitive to the touch. Standing or walking is almost impossible; the sitting or lying position relieves, in favoring the inflamed organs. The bladder and the rectum become, also, sensitive, rendering evacuations from either difficult and painful. During the attack, the fever is accompanied by thirst, a furred tongue, headache, hot skin and nausea. Acute inflammation of the uterus may be confounded with inflammation of the bladder; the physician is the only person qualified to make a differential diagnosis, and therefore should be called to examine the case.

Chronic inflammation of the uterus is more common than the acute; it may be a consequence of an anterior acute attack, but more generally it is the result of continued local irritations. This inflammation is partial rather than general; that is, it occupies a portion of the womb rather than its whole body, and the part more generally affected is the neck. The symptoms of the chronic form vary from the acute, in being much less intense and in the absence of fever. The patient generally experiences a constant dull, aching, deep-seated pain in the lower part of the abdomen, particularly in the groins; also a sensation of weight in front, and a dull, aching pain in the back. The backache is almost constant. Walking, riding, driving, going down stairs, aggravate all these symptoms, and cause the patient to long for rest. Before and during menstruation the pains are greatly increased. The stomach sympathizes in very high degree, and is nauseated at the slightest provocation. The whole system is irritated, inducing repeated sick headaches and various forms of dyspepsia or hysteria. Many cases of dyspepsia and hysteria have been permanently relieved by successfully treating a chronic inflammation of the neck of the womb. In fact, continued nausea, when there is no disease of the stomach, may be taken as a sure sign of chronic inflammation of the womb.

Women thus affected are generally sallow, languid, very sensitive, and liable to headaches, want of appetite, and constipation. Common symptoms complained of by such sufferers are flatulence, heartburn, loss of appetite, foul tongue, constipation, headaches, disordered vision, sleeplessness, bad dreams, flushing of the face, palpitation of the heart, etc.

This form of inflammation is liable to perpetuate itself unless skillfully treated by a physician, as, when long-continued, ulcerations of the neck of the womb are apt to follow, with or without discharge. When the ulcers are very active, or even indolent, discharges occur, which vary from a healthy to a thin, serous, purulent character; they may be so slight as to go unnoticed, or may be very abundant and troublesome. This discharge should not be confounded with leucorrhœa; in ulcerations it is generally of a bloody or of a purulent character; red, yellow, or greenish.

We could not follow in this work the manifold symptoms of structural disorganization resulting from these inflammations; it is a subject on which volumes have been written by very able authors, and one which is more applicable to married women or those advanced in years, than to young unmarried ladies. These diseases are noticed here because they are often the consequences of the simpler disorders of the uterine functions unobserved or neglected in the earlier period of life, when, from ignorance of the functions peculiar to their sex, girls commit acts of indiscretion that eventually lead to the development of such diseases. The several chapters on the various disorders of menstruation should be to them a sufficient guide in the *prevention* of structural diseases. When those diseases appear, no false modesty should prevent their appealing to a skillful physician for aid, as without it years of suffering, and possibly a painful death, will ensue.

DISPLACEMENTS.

An unnatural position of the womb is a disorder which should not affect girls; yet we regret to say that in the higher classes of society it prevails. By referring to the chapter on the anatomy of the womb it will be seen that it is held in place by ligaments, and by the surrounding pressure of the vagina, and other tissues. If, therefore, the condition of a girl is that of general weakness, the ligaments and other tissues are relaxed, and the womb allowed to fall downwards for want of support; this would be a simple case of *prolapsus*, falling of the womb. There are other causes predisposing to this displacement, as: *increased weight and size of the uterus*, which is possible after repeated inflammations, or by the presence of tumors within its chamber; *distention of the abdomen*, induced by habitual constipation, inflammation of the intestines, dropsy, a distended bladder, enlargement of the ovaries, etc.; *pressure on the abdomen*, from tight dresses, corsets, or heavy clothing carried on the hips etc.; *leucorrhœa*, facilitating local weakness and relaxation.

Displacements may, however, occur instantaneously from a great exertion in carrying weights, lifting, straining in defecation or urination; from a leap, a fall on feet or knees, a blow; from long standing, or excessive dancing; from spasmodic coughs, sneezing, and vomiting.

These displacements have received different names according to their character; for the womb may fall forward or backward, or double upon itself. We mention these varieties simply to convey a general idea of their nature and causes. When it falls directly downwards it is called *prolapsus;* when it bends forward, *anteversion;* when backward, *retroversion;* when it bends upon itself forward, *anteflexion;* when it bends upon itself backward, *retroflexion;* and when it projects out of the mouth of the vagina, *procidentia*. There is another, but very rare, variety termed *inversion*, when the fundus of the womb falls within its own cavity.

Bearing in mind the anatomical fact that the womb lies between the bladder and the rectum, it is easily comprehended that if the bladder is kept distended with urine it will press the womb backward upon the rectum; and, *vice versa,* if the rectum is allowed to become unusually distended with fecal matter, it will thrust the womb forward upon the bladder. When this is allowed to go on habitually, the womb acquires that position thus forced upon it, and retains it permanently unless replaced in proper position.

Simple displacements may be carried a long time without causing discomfort, particularly by strong women of a phlegmatic temperament, or of a not very susceptible nervous system; but others, more irritable, soon become aware of some derangement by the innumerable unpleasant sensations of which they become the victims.

The general symptoms are: languor, lassitude, and weakness; the patient is inclined to lie down after every little exertion; there is disposition to pain in the head, in the eyes, temples, and almost constantly in the back; if of nervous temperament, the patient becomes irritable, peevish, excitable and restless; the appetite is very often disturbed, and the stomach often feels as if caving in. The patient is better in the morning, and always after long rest; her feet are cold, and her face often flushed.

The local symptoms are: sensations of fullness, of pressure and of weight in the lower portion of the pelvis; if the womb falls forward, the pressure on the bladder induces a desire to pass water frequently, sometimes with inability to do so; if the womb falls backward, the sensation of pressure and weight is at the rectum. During an evacuation, particularly if constipated, a sensation is felt as if everything were dragged out. "Bearing down" is another and very common sensation, accompanied often by what women thus affected call an "open feeling" at the mouth of the vagina. Standing, walking or riding aggravate all these sensations, while the recumbent position relieves them greatly.

Menstruation is generally regular and painless, unless the womb is bent upon itself, in which case all the symptoms of dysmenorrhœa may be present.

A diagnosis of displacements is not possible from the symptoms above indicated. When there is a suspicion of such an occurrence, a local examination is necessary to determine the case.

These deviations of the position of the uterus are not generally attended with danger; but *if allowed to continue,* the system gradually sympathizes, and we then have an array of unpleasant symptoms never to be relieved until the uterus is properly replaced. Complete rest on the back for a week or two is often sufficient for the uterus to return to its place, provided the obstructions to its accomplishment are removed. When rest is not sufficient to restore it to its place, complications may be expected which only a competent physician should be allowed to treat.

It should be observed here that, although simple displacements may be of little importance to an unmarried woman, they are always grave to a married one; and that, therefore, no young woman should be permitted to remain in such a condition when entering the connubial state.

Having fulfilled a task conceived from many years of experience in the treatment of these diseases, and suggested by an earnest desire to improve the general health of girls, that they may be strong in the fulfillment of their high duties as women, we rest here, conscious that, if we have succeeded in our intent, no greater service could have been rendered to that sex in which man finds mother, wife, and daughter; and all the endearments and pleasures which give to life its chief joy, happiness and comfort.

$18\frac{1}{2}$

INDEX.

A.

	PAGE
ACCIDENTS, what they teach	26
ADOLESCENCE	73
AIR, in relation to human health	173
Hot and *Dry*, effects of, upon health	173
Cold and *Dry*	174
Damp and *Hot*	176
Cold and *Humid*	176
In *Motion*	177
Mountain	178
Sea	179
Temperature of	180
Rapid changes of the	180
Of dwellings	180
Causes of bad, of dwellings	180
Change of, or ventilation	180
How affected by noxious gases in dwellings	181
Of the sick room	186
Affecting girls at school	187
AMENORRHOEA	218
Delayed Menstruation.	
Causes of	219
Treatment of	220
Suppressed Menstruation.	
Causes of	221
Treatment of	226
Retained Menstruation.	
Causes of	228
Treatment of	230
ATMOSPHERE (*see Air*).	
A VEXED QUESTION	16

B.

BEAUMONT's experiments on the digestibility of Food	129-146
BILE, its function in digestion	128

	PAGE
BLOOD, Circulation of	135
Purification of	138
BONES of woman, and of man	37
BOYS AND GIRLS, their mode of growth, morally and physically	19-31
BREASTS, anatomy and physiology of	52
Necessity for well-developed	53
Dress in relation to the growth of	53
Hygiene to secure a good development of	54
Of woman, and of man	36

C.

CATALEPSY, distinguished from Hysteria (see *Hysteria*).	
CHEMISTRY and digestion	137
CHEST of woman and of man	38
CHYME	127
CHYLE	127
CHLOROSIS	230
Symptoms of	231
Cause of	231
Treatment of	231
CIRCLE OF LIFE	138
CITY LIFE, dangers of	67-68
CLOTHING in relation to the preservation of the life of girls	152
Heat-conducting power of *Linen*	154
" " *Flax*	154
" " *Cotton*	154
" " *Wool*	154
" " *Silk*	154
" " *Fur*	154
" " *Feathers*	154
Electrical conducting power of	154

	PAGE
CLOTHING, *Shape* of	155
Corset as an article of	156
Color of	157
The head	158
The neck	159
The trunk	159
The extremities	160
Reflections upon	163
Constipation from partial	168
Emblematic	170
Should be equally warm all over	163
COTTON, heat conducting power of	154
CORSET, as an article of dress	156
History of the	156
Baneful effects of the	156
COLOR OF CLOTHING in relation to heat	157
CONSTIPATION, from unequal dressing	168
The cause of displacements of the womb	169-170
CRISIS, Menstrual, commencement and natural course	85-92

D.

DANCING, effect of, on health	118
DEMENTIA	74
DIGESTION, process of	128
DISPLACEMENTS of the womb (see *Womb*).	
DRESSING (see *Clothing*).	
DRIVING, effect of, on health	120
DYSMENORRHOEA	241
Painful Menstruation.	
Causes of	242-244
Symptoms of	243
Simple	245
Accidental	246
Congestive	246
Inflammatory	246
Mechanical or physical	247
Treatment of	248

E.

ELECTRICITY, conducting power of, by various articles of clothing	154

	PAGE
EPILEPSY, distinguished from Hysteria (see *Hysteria*).	
EQUALITY of the Sexes, to be one of excellence, not kind	23
EXERCISE, and its relation to bodily functions	114
Walking	117
Riding	117
Dancing	118
Rowing	120
Games	120
Driving	120
Sea-going	121
Singing	122
Of girls at school	123
EXTREMITIES, clothing of the	160

F.

FALLOPIAN TUBES, their anatomy, functions, and position in pelvis	49
FASHION, as a social law	102-109
Its exaggerations	110
FEATHERS, heat conducting power of	154
FLAX, heat conducting power of	154
FOOD, and its relation to the preservation of life	125
Beaumont's experiments on the digestibility of various articles of food	129-146
As classified by Liebig	130
And its progress in civilization	130
And chemistry	136
Adaptation of the elements of, to the want of the body	142
Proportionate elements of (table)	142
Respiratory	144
Nitrogenized	144
As affecting character	148
Rules for taking	149-151
FUNCTIONAL IRREGULARITIES OF MENSTRUATION	190
Symptoms of	192
Regimen to be observed in	193
Predisposing Causes of	197
Temperaments	88
Diet	197-199

	PAGE
Bad Air	200
Want of Exercise	200
Over Study	201-209
Exposure	209
Pressure	209
Uncleanliness	210
Idleness	210
Immediate Causes of,	
Exposure to sudden change	212
Emotions	212
Love	216
Accidents, &c.	217
Fur, heat conducting power of	154

G.

Games, effects of, on health	120
Gases, noxious gases in dwellings.	181
From burning coal	183
" " wood	183
" " oil	184
" " candles	184
Illuminating	183
Dangerous, from water-closets and stationary basins	185
Gastric Juice, function of the, in digestion	126
Girls and Boys, their mode of growth, morally and physically	19-31
At school	187
Green Sickness	230
Symptoms of	231
Causes of	232
Treatment of	232

H.

Head, clothing of the	158
Health in the struggle for existence	21
And Vigor, the foundations for success in life	24
What is?	26
Violation of the laws of, and human responsibility regarding it	26-27

	PAGE
Hemorrhage, distinguished from Menorrhagia (see *Menorrhagia*).	
Hygienic Generalities: Air, Food, Light and Exercise	95-99
Hysteria	258
Causes of	260
Distinguished from Catalepsy.	264
" " Epilepsy .	264
Diseases simulated by	264
Symptoms of	266
Treatment of	269

I.

Ice-Water and Ices	129
Ignorance, and its effects on health	9
Imagination, influence of, on hastening puberty	87
Mind and	201
Infancy	73
Inflammation of the Womb (see *Womb*).	

K.

Knowledge of the body	17

L.

Leucorrhoea	251
Causes of	252
Symptoms of	253
Acute	254
Chronic	254
Transient	255
Intermittent	255
Treatment of	256
Liebig's classification of food	130
Limbs of woman and of man	37
Linen, heat conducting power of.	154

M.

Man's superior advantages over woman the result of physical superiority in power	21

INDEX.

	PAGE
MAN and woman the complement of each other	23
And woman physically compared in growth	31-39
Reasons for his leadership	24
MENORRHAGIA	234

Excessive Menstruation.

Causes of	236
Distinguished from hemorrhage	237
Active	238
Passive	238
Nervous	238
Spasmodic	238
Treatment of	238
MENSTRUATION: Physiological process	75-78
Warning symptoms	76
As related to ovulation	79-85
Of city and of country girls	86-87
Affected by excitement, education, temperament	88
Duration of	88
Reappearance of, after suspension	89
Natural disturbances of	91
(See *Puberty*)	75
Delayed (see *Amenorrhœa*).	
Epoch of its commencement and mode of its course	75-92
Suppression of (see *Amenorrhœa*).	
Retention of (see *Amenorrhœa*).	
Chlorotic (see *Amenorrhœa*).	
Excessive (see *Menorrhagia*).	
Painful (see *Dysmenorrhœa*).	
Periodicity	80
General irregularities of	190
Functional irregularity of	191
Symptoms of	192
Regimen	193
Causes of	197
" immediate	210
" accidental	211
MODESTY, of timidity	12
True	13
MOTHERS, Duty of	7
Appeal to, to instruct daughters in functions of their sex	13-14
Sad story	204
MUSCLES of woman and of man	37

N.

NECK, clothing of the	159

O.

OVARIES, their anatomy and position in pelvis	41
Functions	41-49
OVULATION as connected with Menstruation	80-85

P.

PANCREATIC JUICE, its function in digestion	128
PELVIS, anatomy of	40
In relation to woman's safety	40
Difference of, in the two sexes	42
Growth of	43
How to preserve its proportions	42
Advice to mothers for the protection of the, in girls	44
PHYSIOLOGY as a moral teacher	26-30
PUBERTY	70
Menstruation the characteristic of, in woman	75
Warning symptoms of, in young girls	76-78

R.

RESPONSIBILITY of parents and teachers	10
RIDING, effects of, on health	117
ROWING, effects of, on health	120

S.

SALIVA, function of, in digestion	126
SCHOOL, exercise for girls at	123
Houses, air of, affecting girls	187
SEA-GOING, effects of, on health	121
SEA-SICKNESS, how to avoid, effects of, on health	121

INDEX.

Sexes, moral and physical difference of the 31
Shape of Clothing in relation to the maintenance of animal heat 155
Silk, heat conducting power of .. 154
Singing, effect of, on health 122
Skin, its part in nutrition 126
Society in its relations to the health of girls 100-113
Social law 101
Social Excitement and its consequences — experience of Georges Sand 111-112
Stature of woman and of man .. 36
Symptoms of Menstrual disturbance,
   Normal 91
   Abnormal 190-196

T.

Temperaments 59
   Knowledge of, necessary 59
   Sanguine, and its hygiene ... 61
   Lymphatic, and its hygiene .. 62
   Bilious, and its hygiene 64
   Nervous, and its hygiene 65
   Mixed, etc. 66
Temperature of the body as affected by dress 152-154
   Evil results of unequal ..167-170

Trunk, clothing of the 159

V.

Virility 73
Vital Force and digestion 137

W.

Walking, effects of on health ... 117
Whites (see *Leucorrhœa*).
Woman's Strength in relation to occupation 22
Woman and Man the complement of each other 23
   Her moral and physical characteristics 31-33
   Necessity of her self-knowledge 11-14
Womb, position of 41
   Anatomy of 46
   Its growth 48
   Inflammation of 274
   Displacement of 274
   Symptoms of inflammation of. 275
   Causes of inflammation of ... 275
   Symptoms and causes of displacement of 278-280
Wool, heat conducting power of.. 154